To my incredible husband, for embracing this journey with me, and to our amazing children, whose unwavering support and endless encouragement keep us grounded and inspired.

Here's to more years filled with good health, happiness and plenty of adventures.
Allison x

From Blaming Myself to Finding the Truth: How Intermittent Fasting Changed My Life

Allison Butnick

Table of Contents

Disclaimer

The content of this book, ***"From Blaming Myself to Finding the Truth: How Intermittent Fasting Changed My Life"*** is intended for informational and educational purposes only. The insights and experiences shared are based on my personal journey with intermittent fasting and are not intended as professional medical or nutritional advice.

I am not a qualified medical practitioner, nutritionist, or dietitian. The information provided herein is drawn from my own experiences and research. While I strive to provide accurate and up-to-date information, there may be errors or omissions, and individual results can vary.

Before starting any new dietary regimen, including intermittent fasting, it is essential to consult with a healthcare professional. This is especially important if you have pre-existing health conditions, are pregnant, nursing, or taking any medications. A medical professional can provide personalised advice based on your unique health needs and circumstances.

The strategies and recommendations discussed in this book are not meant to replace professional medical advice, diagnosis, or treatment. Always seek the advice of your physician or other qualified health provider with any questions you may have regarding a medical condition or dietary change.

I am not responsible for any adverse effects or consequences resulting from the use of any of the suggestions, techniques, or recommendations mentioned in this book. Your health and well-being are paramount, and it is crucial to make informed decisions in consultation with your healthcare provider.

Thank you for reading and I wish you success along your journey to better health.

Chapter 1: Introduction

How it Started

At 55, having dedicated much of my life to understanding nutrition, I found myself grappling with a persistent struggle: weight management. Though not extreme, the extra two stone (28lbs) I carried was increasingly noticeable and disheartening. My youthful ability to lose weight quickly through short-term measures no longer worked, and decades of trying various diets left me feeling defeated and frustrated.

In 2002, as my wedding approached, I embarked on an Atkins-style diet—high in protein and fat, low in carbs. Despite my best efforts, after several months of sticking to the very restrictive regime, all I had lost was the will to live and a measly five pounds. This arduous journey left me feeling thoroughly depressed; I blamed myself for the lack of progress.

As the years passed and life grew more demanding with raising children and managing daily stress, my weight challenges persisted. Despite cooking healthy meals and adopting a low-carb approach, I found myself stuck in a cycle of minimal weight loss, which was often only achievable through severe calorie restrictions. My attempts at regular exercise, from running to yoga, offered some health benefits but failed to address the root issue of my weight.

Everything changed in August 2023 when I stumbled upon the insights of Dr. Mindy Pelz, Chris van Tulleken and Davinia Taylor. Their perspectives on intermittent fasting, ultra processed foods and understanding the impact of hormones on everything we do, resonated deeply, leading me to explore their incredible books and podcasts. For the first time, I gained clarity on how our bodies truly utilise energy—how our brains prefer stored fat over readily available food energy, and how continuous food consumption disrupts this natural balance.

Intrigued by these revelations, my husband and I decided to implement intermittent fasting. Building up to a narrowed eating window from 4 pm to 8 pm daily, we gradually introduced longer fasts, including 36-hour and 48-hour fasts, eventually pushing to a 72-hour fast. Remarkably, the results were transformative.

Within a month, we noticed significant health improvements and after a few weeks of adjustment, weirdly, neither of us felt hungry, dizzy or deprived of food, even though we were consuming way less than we had been conditioned to think we needed. No longer were we constantly planning the next meal; we dropped the construct of breakfast being the most important meal of the day (interestingly this originally came from Dr. John Harvey Kellogg, the inventor of corn flakes); never thought about calorie counting, weighing our food, or ourselves; and the idea of three meals a day became a dim and distant memory!

Now, less than a year later, I've lost over two stone, and my husband has shed more than three (42lbs). I'm fitting into clothes from my early 20's and feeling revitalised. This journey has shown me that achieving sustainable health can be simpler than I imagined—without the hunger, irritability, and minimal results of past diets.

Why I Wrote This Book

This book is a reflection on my transformative experience with intermittent fasting—a method that not only changed my approach to health but also delivered results, fast. My goal is to share this life-changing approach with others who, like me, have faced persistent weight challenges.

I will take you through the principles of intermittent fasting, explain the science behind why it works, and provide practical advice on how to incorporate it into your daily routine effectively, adopting a balanced, nourishing approach to eating that goes beyond mere weight loss. You'll also learn about the key lifestyle changes that complemented our fasting journey.

My hope is that this story inspires you to discover a path to health that is both sustainable and truly life enhancing.

Chapter 2: My Background and Struggles

When I look back at my life, I can see how my relationship with food and my body has evolved over the years. Like many people, my struggle with weight and health didn't happen overnight—it was a gradual build-up of habits, challenges, and life circumstances that brought me to where I am today.

Early Life and Dieting History

Growing up, I was always conscious of my weight. My family valued healthy eating, and I learned early on the importance of fruits, vegetables, and home-cooked meals. However, despite these good habits, I was never one of those people who could eat whatever they wanted without gaining weight. As a teenager, I was already aware of the concept of dieting, although my knowledge at the time was limited to whatever fad diet was popular in the magazines.

My 20's and 30's were a rollercoaster of trying different diets. I've tried everything—from low-fat diets to calorie counting, to cutting out carbs completely. There were moments of success, where I managed to lose some weight, but it always came back, often with a little extra. I became increasingly frustrated and disheartened, questioning why nothing seemed to work long-term.

The Impact of Aging on Weight and Health

As I entered my 40's, the struggle intensified. The combination of work, raising a family, and the natural aging process made weight loss even more challenging. My metabolism wasn't what it used to be, and the energy I once had to exercise regularly was often sapped by the demands of daily life. Even though I was eating what I thought was a healthy diet, the pounds were creeping on, and it became harder and harder to lose them.

The changes in my body were not just about weight gain. I started noticing other signs of aging—my energy levels were lower, I was more prone to digestive issues, aching joints and my sleep was often restless. My body was sending me signals that something needed to change, but I wasn't sure what that change was.
During this time, I tried to stay active. I walked regularly, attended exercise classes, and made sure to eat plenty of fruit and vegetables. But no matter how much effort I put into staying healthy, I always felt like I was fighting an uphill battle. The persistent weight gain and my increasing frustration made me feel trapped in a cycle I couldn't break. **It's true, you can't outrun a bad diet!**

The Emotional Toll of the Struggle

It wasn't just the physical changes that were hard to cope with; the emotional toll was just as significant. Every time I tried a new diet or exercise regimen, I was filled with hope—only to be let down when the results didn't match my expectations. I felt like I was constantly failing, despite my best efforts. This cycle of hope and disappointment took a toll on my self-esteem. I began to internalise the belief that no matter what I did, I would never truly be healthy or comfortable in my own skin.

I also became more self-conscious about how others saw me. Social gatherings became a source of anxiety—what if someone commented on my weight? I found myself avoiding situations where food was the focus because I didn't want to be judged for what I was eating or not eating. This anxiety only added to the stress and made me feel even more isolated.

The Turning Point

By the time I reached my 50's, I was desperate for a change. I knew that I needed to do something different—something sustainable that could bring back my energy, help me lose weight, and restore my confidence. But after years of trying and failing, I wasn't sure where to turn. I felt like I had exhausted every option.

This was the backdrop to my eventual discovery of intermittent fasting. Looking back, I can see how my entire journey, with all its ups and downs, was preparing me for this moment. My years of trial and error taught me one thing: true, lasting change doesn't come from quick fixes or extreme measures. It comes from understanding your body, listening to its needs, and finding a way to work with it rather than against it.

In the chapters that follow, I will share how intermittent fasting became that sustainable change for me, transforming not just my body but my entire approach to health and well-being.

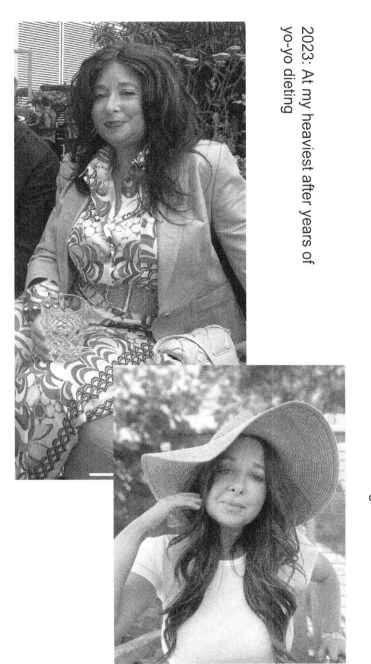

2023: At my heaviest after years of yo-yo dieting

2024: After less than a year following Intermittent Fasting

Chapter 3: The Moment of Change

Breaking Free from Flawed Food Myths

As I reflect on my journey to better health, one stark realisation stands out: ***much of the conventional wisdom around food and nutrition that I grew up with was deeply flawed.*** The education we received from health authorities, governments, and even well-meaning experts was often misguided. It led many of us down a path that, instead of promoting health, contributed to the very problems we were trying to avoid.

For decades, we were told that fat was the enemy. "Low-fat" became the mantra of a generation. Products proudly displayed their "low-fat" labels as if they were the key to health, while fats—especially saturated fats—were demonised. We were encouraged to shun foods like eggs, butter, and red meat in favour of carbohydrate-laden, highly processed alternatives. What we didn't realise was that, in stripping these foods of their natural fats, manufacturers were replacing them with sugars, artificial sweeteners, and unhealthy oils to make them palatable.

This shift, now widely recognised as a significant mistake, had unintended consequences. The reduction of healthy fats in our diets coincided with an increase in refined carbohydrates and sugars, leading to a cascade of metabolic issues. We were told to avoid cholesterol-rich foods like eggs, despite their nutritional benefits, and to limit meat consumption without understanding the differences between processed meats and grass-fed, organic options.

Simultaneously, the rise of vegetable oils like sunflower oil, rape seed oil, and corn oil—heavily processed and rich in inflammatory omega-6 fatty acids—further exacerbated the problem. These oils were marketed as "heart-healthy" alternatives to traditional fats, yet they contributed to chronic inflammation, obesity, and a host of other health issues.

This broader trend towards processed foods is meticulously explored in Dr. Chris van Tulleken's book, *Ultra-Processed People*. Van Tulleken delves into how the industrial food industry has reshaped our diets, filling our grocery stores with ultra-processed foods (UPFs) designed to be addictive and convenient, but which lack real nutritional value. He explains how these foods, often marketed as healthy or low-fat, have become central to our diets, contributing to the obesity epidemic and numerous health problems. His work highlights how these UPFs manipulate our brains and bodies, driving overeating and fostering dependency on foods that do more harm than good.

Add to this the growing convenience of fast food, the proliferation of takeaway options, and the increasing reliance on ultra-processed foods, and it's no surprise that waistlines expanded, and health declined. Our kitchens became stocked with boxed cereals, frozen meals, and sugary snacks, all of which were designed for convenience, not nutrition.

Another pervasive myth that deserves scrutiny is the notion that calorie counting is a reliable method for long-term weight management. Despite decades of promotion, if calorie counting were an effective and sustainable tool for weight loss, we would see a dramatic reduction in obesity rates and slimming clubs wouldn't have repeat members. The reality is that the body's metabolic processes are far more complex than a simple equation of calories in versus calories out. Factors like hormonal balance, nutrient density, and metabolic health play crucial roles in weight management. Calorie counting often overlooks these complexities, leading to frustration and temporary results rather than lasting change.

Moreover, the advent of new weight loss drugs, such as GLP-1 receptor agonists (e.g., Ozempic and Wegovy), has introduced another layer of controversy. While these medications show promise in aiding weight loss, their long-term effects on health are still largely unknown. Early reports suggest that they can be effective in reducing body weight, but questions remain about their impact on overall health and well-being. The long-term safety of these drugs, their potential side effects, and their effects on metabolic health need further investigation. It is crucial to approach these new treatments with caution and to consider them as part of a broader, more holistic approach to health.

As I educated myself on real, whole foods and the importance of healthy fats, I realised how misled we had been. The food pyramid, with its emphasis on grains and minimal fats, was not a prescription for health but a recipe for disaster. The low-fat era did not make us healthier; it made us hungrier, heavier, and sicker.

By understanding where we went wrong, we can now make more informed choices. The path to health is not paved with processed foods, artificial ingredients, and misguided nutritional advice. Instead, it lies in returning to whole, unprocessed foods—embracing healthy fats, consuming quality proteins, and rejecting the sugar-laden and chemically altered products that have dominated our diets for too long.

It's time to rewrite the narrative, discard the outdated and harmful myths, and reclaim our health with knowledge, balance, and a renewed appreciation for the foods that truly nourish us.

Discovering Intermittent Fasting

In August 2023, my perspective on health and weight management underwent a significant shift. Through watching videos and reading books by Davinia Taylor, and Dr. Mindy Pelz, I discovered intermittent fasting. This chapter recounts how I came across intermittent fasting, the initial scepticism, and the gradual adoption of this new approach.

Key Influencers along the journey

Davinia Taylor and Dr. Mindy Pelz were instrumental in reshaping my understanding of nutrition and fasting. Their insights provided clarity on how intermittent fasting could address my long-standing issues with weight and health. Their work influenced my decision to embrace intermittent fasting, along with the removal of UPFs from my diet.

The Epiphany: Understanding the Science Behind Fasting

Through my exploration of intermittent fasting, I came to understand the science behind it—how our bodies utilise stored fat for energy, the impact of frequent food consumption on insulin levels, and the benefits of allowing the body to fast. This section explains the key scientific principles that underpin intermittent fasting, offering insight into why this approach was so effective for me.

How Intermittent Fasting Works: Fasting and the Metabolic Switch

Intermittent fasting is the key to triggering a metabolic switch from using glucose as the primary energy source to using fat. As you fast, your insulin levels drop, and the body begins to break down stored glycogen for energy. Once glycogen is depleted, the body transitions to fat burning, entering a state of ketosis. This switch not only helps with weight loss but also improves metabolic health in a variety of ways:

Autophagy: Cellular Cleanup
Another significant benefit of intermittent fasting is autophagy, a natural process where the body cleans out damaged cells and regenerates new ones. Autophagy is a critical defence mechanism against diseases like cancer, neurodegenerative disorders, and infections. It also plays a role in aging, as it removes dysfunctional proteins and organelles, helping to maintain cellular health.
Autophagy is typically activated during periods of fasting when the body needs to optimise resources. This cellular cleanup contributes to the anti-aging effects of fasting and its potential to enhance longevity.

Impact on Hormones and Longevity

Intermittent fasting also influences other hormones, such as growth hormone, which plays a role in fat loss, muscle gain, and overall vitality. Fasting has been shown to increase growth hormone levels significantly, which supports fat burning and muscle preservation during weight loss.

Moreover, intermittent fasting has been linked to improved longevity. Studies on animals have shown that fasting can extend lifespan by reducing inflammation, improving insulin sensitivity, and enhancing cellular repair processes. While research in humans is ongoing, the potential anti-aging benefits of fasting are promising.

Scientific Evidence Supporting Intermittent Fasting

Weight Loss and Fat Reduction

Several studies have demonstrated the effectiveness of intermittent fasting for weight loss. A review published in *Obesity Reviews* found that intermittent fasting resulted in a 3–8% weight reduction over 3 to 24 weeks. The participants also experienced a significant decrease in waist circumference, indicating a reduction in visceral fat, the harmful fat that surrounds internal organs.

Improved Metabolic Health

Research also shows that intermittent fasting can improve various metabolic markers, including insulin sensitivity, blood pressure, and cholesterol levels. For example, a study in the *Journal of Translational Medicine* found that participants who practiced intermittent fasting had lower fasting insulin levels, reduced insulin resistance, and lower blood pressure compared to those who ate regularly throughout the day.

Brain Health and Cognitive Function
Intermittent fasting may also benefit brain health. Animal studies have shown that fasting enhances the production of brain-derived neurotrophic factor (BDNF), a protein that supports brain function and protects against neurodegenerative diseases like Alzheimer's and Parkinson's. Fasting has also been shown to improve cognitive function and reduce inflammation, which is linked to cognitive decline. Understanding the science behind intermittent fasting helps clarify why it is more than just a weight-loss trend. By leveraging the body's natural processes— such as fat burning, autophagy, and hormone regulation—fasting offers a holistic approach to improving metabolic health, longevity, and overall well-being. In the following sections, I'll share how applying these principles transformed my health and how they can do the same for you.

Chapter 4. Understanding the Body's Energy Sources

To fully grasp the benefits of intermittent fasting, it's important to understand how our bodies source and use energy. In this chapter, we'll explore the processes behind how the body converts food and stored fat into energy, the role of metabolism in weight management, and why traditional diets often fail to deliver sustainable results.

How the Body Uses Food and Stored Fat for Energy

Our bodies require a constant supply of energy to perform everyday functions—from thinking and moving to breathing and digesting. This energy primarily comes from the food we consume, which is broken down into glucose (sugar) and used to fuel our cells.

When we eat, especially carbohydrate-rich foods, our blood sugar levels rise, prompting the pancreas to release insulin. Insulin helps transport glucose from the bloodstream into cells, where it's either used immediately for energy or stored as glycogen in the liver and muscles. Glycogen is the body's short-term energy reserve, and it's highly accessible when quick energy is needed, such as during physical activity or between meals. However, the body's glycogen storage capacity is limited—once these stores are full, any excess glucose is converted into fat and stored in adipose tissue for long-term energy.

During periods when we're not eating, such as overnight or between meals, the body starts to draw on these glycogen reserves. If the fasting period is extended, such as with intermittent fasting, the glycogen stores in the liver are depleted. At this point, the body switches to using stored fat as its primary energy source. This transition is a key aspect of intermittent fasting, as it allows the body to tap into fat reserves more effectively, promoting weight loss and metabolic health.

The Role of Metabolism

Metabolism encompasses all the chemical reactions in the body that convert food into energy. This process includes two main components: catabolism, where the body breaks down nutrients to release energy, and anabolism, where energy is used to build and repair tissues.

The rate at which your body burns calories—known as your metabolic rate—depends on various factors, including age, muscle mass, activity level, and genetics. A faster metabolism means more calories burned, even at rest, while a slower metabolism burns fewer calories, making weight management more challenging.

Traditional diets typically emphasise reduction to achieve weight loss. While this may work initially, the body often responds by slowing down its metabolism to conserve energy—a survival mechanism rooted in our evolutionary past. This metabolic slowdown can lead to a plateau in weight loss, where progress stalls, and regaining lost weight becomes almost inevitable once the diet ends.

Why Traditional Diets Often Fail

Many traditional diets focus on cutting calories or specific food groups without considering how the body's energy systems work. While these diets can result in short-term weight loss, they often fail in the long run due to several factors:

1. **Metabolic Adaptation:** When calorie intake is reduced, the body adapts by lowering its metabolic rate, making further weight loss more difficult and increasing the likelihood of weight regain.

2. **Glycogen Depletion and Hunger:** Calorie-restricted diets often lead to the rapid depletion of glycogen stores, which can trigger intense hunger and cravings. Once glycogen is depleted, many diets fail to provide a sustainable way to transition into burning fat, leading to feelings of deprivation and eventual overeating.

3. **Insulin Resistance:** Frequent eating, particularly of high-carb or processed foods, can lead to insulin resistance. This condition reduces the body's ability to efficiently manage blood sugar levels, making it harder to lose weight and increasing the risk of chronic health issues like type 2 diabetes.

4. **Lack of Flexibility:** Many diets are rigid, requiring strict adherence to specific foods or eating schedules. This lack of flexibility can make it challenging to sustain the diet long-term, especially when faced with the realities of a busy lifestyle.

Intermittent fasting addresses these issues by allowing the body to deplete its glycogen stores and naturally transition into burning stored fat for energy.

By extending the fasting period, the body is encouraged to access fat reserves more consistently, leading to more sustainable weight loss and improved metabolic health. **Unlike traditional diets, intermittent fasting doesn't focus on what you eat, but rather when you eat**, offering a more flexible and natural approach to achieving long-term health goals.

In the following chapters, we'll dive into the practical aspects of implementing intermittent fasting and explore the various methods you can use to tailor this approach to your lifestyle.

Chapter 5. The Role of Insulin and Blood Sugar

The Science of Blood Sugar and Insulin

Insulin: The Fat-Storing Hormone

Insulin is a crucial hormone produced by the pancreas that regulates blood sugar levels and influences how our bodies manage energy. Its primary function is to facilitate the uptake of glucose from the bloodstream into cells, where it can be used for energy. However, insulin also plays a significant role in fat metabolism.

When you consume a carbohydrate-rich meal, your blood sugar levels rise, prompting the pancreas to release insulin. This surge in insulin helps cells absorb glucose, but it also inhibits the breakdown of fat. Essentially, insulin signals the body to prioritise glucose as an immediate energy source, thereby suppressing fat burning. As a result, the body stores excess glucose as fat, leading to weight gain if this cycle is repeated frequently.

In today's world, many diets are high in refined sugars and processed foods, which can cause frequent spikes in insulin levels. This constant elevation in insulin prevents the body from accessing stored fat for energy and promotes the accumulation of fat tissue. Over time, this can lead to a condition known as **insulin resistance**, where the body's cells become less responsive to insulin's effects.

The Link Between Insulin Resistance and Chronic Diseases

Insulin resistance is a condition where the body's cells no longer respond effectively to insulin. As a result, the pancreas produces more insulin to try to compensate for this decreased sensitivity. Initially, this compensatory mechanism can maintain normal blood sugar levels, but over time, it can lead to elevated insulin levels in the blood, known as **hyperinsulinemia.**

This condition is a precursor to type 2 diabetes and is associated with several other serious health issues, including:

- **Obesity**: Elevated insulin levels promote fat storage, particularly around the abdominal area. This contributes to weight gain and obesity, which further exacerbates insulin resistance.
- **Heart Disease**: Chronic insulin resistance is linked to an increased risk of heart disease. Elevated insulin levels can lead to inflammation, higher blood pressure, and increased cholesterol levels, all of which are risk factors for cardiovascular problems.
- **Metabolic Syndrome**: Insulin resistance is a key component of metabolic syndrome, a cluster of conditions that includes high blood pressure, high blood sugar, excess abdominal fat, and abnormal cholesterol levels. This syndrome increases the risk of type 2 diabetes, heart disease, and stroke.
- **Fatty Liver Disease**: Insulin resistance can lead to the accumulation of fat in the liver, resulting in non-alcoholic fatty liver disease

(NAFLD). This condition can progress to non-alcoholic steatohepatitis (NASH) and even cirrhosis if left untreated.
- **Hormonal Imbalances**: Insulin resistance can disrupt the balance of other hormones in the body, including those related to reproductive health. This can lead to conditions such as polycystic ovary syndrome (PCOS) in women, which affects menstrual cycles and fertility.

Managing Insulin Resistance Through Diet and Lifestyle

1. **Reducing Meal Frequency:**
   Intermittent Fasting: One effective strategy to manage insulin levels is intermittent fasting. By reducing the frequency of meals and extending periods between eating, insulin levels can drop, allowing the body to use stored fat for energy more efficiently. This approach also gives the pancreas a break from constant insulin production, improving overall insulin sensitivity.
2. **Choosing Low-Glycaemic Foods:**
   Whole Foods: Incorporating whole, unprocessed foods into your diet can help stabilise blood sugar levels. Foods with a low glycaemic index (GI) release glucose slowly into the bloodstream, preventing rapid spikes in insulin levels.
   High Fibre Foods: Foods high in fibre, such as fruits, vegetables, legumes, and whole grains, help slow the absorption of glucose and improve blood sugar control.
3. **Food Order Matters**

The *"Glucose Goddess"* approach, popularised by biochemist Jessie Inchauspé, offers a practical and science-backed way to manage blood sugar levels by strategically choosing the order in which you eat your food. Jessie's work focuses on simple yet effective methods to flatten glucose spikes, improve energy, and reduce cravings, all without cutting out entire food groups.

One of the key principles of the 'Glucose Goddess' method is to **always start your meal with a serving of vegetables**. This isn't just about eating more greens; it's about harnessing the power of fibre. When you eat fibre-rich vegetables first, the fibre forms a gel-like substance in your stomach that slows down the absorption of sugars and starches from the rest of your meal. This results in a more gradual rise in blood sugar, keeping insulin levels stable and preventing the sharp spikes that can lead to energy crashes and cravings.

By applying this approach, you can still enjoy your favourite foods—pasta, bread, even desserts—without the negative effects of blood sugar spikes. The key is to always eat your vegetables first. This simple habit can lead to significant improvements in metabolic health, weight management, and even mental clarity.

Incorporating the Glucose Goddess strategy into your intermittent fasting routine enhances its effectiveness. By controlling glucose and insulin levels, you maintain more stable energy throughout your fasting period and reduce the intensity of hunger pangs. This approach makes your meals more satisfying, further supporting your overall health goals while allowing you to enjoy high-quality, nutrient-dense foods.

4. **Incorporating Healthy Fats and Proteins:**
   Healthy Fats: Including sources of healthy fats, such as avocados, nuts, seeds, and olive oil, can help stabilise insulin levels and support overall metabolic health.
   Lean Proteins: Consuming lean proteins, such as chicken, fish, tofu, and legumes, can aid in maintaining muscle mass and promote satiety, reducing the likelihood of excessive snacking and insulin spikes.

5. **Regular Physical Activity:**
   Exercise: Engaging in regular physical activity improves insulin sensitivity and helps the body use glucose more effectively. Both aerobic exercises (such as walking, running, or cycling) and resistance training (such as weightlifting) are beneficial.

6. **Avoiding Processed Foods and Sugars:**
   Minimising Refined Carbohydrates: Reducing the intake of processed foods and sugary beverages can help lower insulin levels and reduce the risk of developing insulin resistance. Focus on whole, nutrient-dense foods that provide lasting energy without causing blood sugar spikes.

The Benefits of Improved Insulin Sensitivity

Improving insulin sensitivity through dietary and lifestyle changes can have a profound impact on overall health. Enhanced insulin sensitivity means that the body can more effectively manage blood sugar levels, reduce fat storage, and lower the risk of developing type 2 diabetes and other metabolic disorders. Additionally, improved insulin sensitivity contributes to better energy levels, reduced inflammation, and a lower risk of cardiovascular disease.

Understanding the role of insulin and blood sugar management is crucial for maintaining a healthy weight and preventing and in some cases even reversing chronic diseases. By adopting strategies such as intermittent fasting, choosing low-glycaemic foods, incorporating healthy fats and proteins, engaging in regular exercise, and avoiding processed foods, you can effectively manage insulin levels and improve overall health.

These changes not only support better insulin sensitivity but also contribute to a more balanced and sustainable approach to health and well-being. As always, consult with a healthcare professional before making significant changes to your diet or lifestyle, especially if you have pre-existing health conditions.

Chapter 6: Understanding and Managing Inflammation

The Havoc of Inflammation on Our Bodies

Inflammation is a vital response of the immune system to injury, infection, or harmful stimuli, characterised by redness, heat, swelling, and pain. While acute inflammation is a normal part of the healing process, chronic inflammation is a different story. It's a persistent, low-level inflammation that can cause significant damage over time and is linked to numerous health issues.

Chronic inflammation can disrupt normal bodily functions, contributing to various diseases and conditions. It's not just a standalone issue but a complex factor that exacerbates other health problems. Understanding its role and managing it effectively is crucial for maintaining overall health.

How Inflammation Manifests Through Different Diseases

Inflammation can have widespread effects, manifesting in various diseases and conditions:

- **Cardiovascular Disease**: Chronic inflammation contributes to atherosclerosis, where plaque builds up in the arteries, leading to heart attacks, strokes, and other cardiovascular issues.
- **Type 2 Diabetes**: Persistent inflammation impairs insulin sensitivity, leading to insulin resistance and contributing to type 2 diabetes. This disruption affects blood sugar regulation and can exacerbate other health problems.

- **Arthritis**: Conditions like rheumatoid arthritis and osteoarthritis are characterised by joint inflammation, leading to pain, stiffness, and reduced mobility.
- **Autoimmune Diseases**: In autoimmune disorders such as lupus and multiple sclerosis, the immune system erroneously attacks healthy tissues, causing chronic inflammation and tissue damage.
- **Cancer**: Chronic inflammation is linked to an increased risk of developing certain cancers. Inflammatory processes can create an environment that supports tumour growth and spread.
- **Glaucoma**: Chronic inflammation in the eye can contribute to increased intraocular pressure, which is a risk factor for glaucoma. Managing inflammation is crucial to prevent damage to the optic nerve and preserve vision.
- **Fatty Liver Disease**: Inflammation plays a significant role in non-alcoholic fatty liver disease (NAFLD). Persistent inflammation in the liver can lead to fatty accumulation, liver damage, and potentially progress to non-alcoholic steatohepatitis (NASH) or cirrhosis.
- **Skin Problems**: Conditions such as acne, eczema, and psoriasis are often linked to chronic inflammation. Managing inflammation can help reduce flare-ups and improve skin health.
- **Fertility Issues**: Chronic inflammation can impact reproductive health, potentially affecting fertility in both men and women. In women, inflammation may disrupt hormonal balance and impair ovarian function, while in men, it can affect sperm quality and quantity.

Reducing Inflammation Through Lowering Blood Sugar and Insulin Spikes

Managing inflammation involves addressing factors that contribute to its persistence. One effective strategy is stabilising blood sugar levels and reducing insulin spikes, as these are closely related to inflammation.

1. **Lowering Blood Sugar Levels:**
   o Balanced Diet: Opt for a diet rich in whole foods, such as fruits, vegetables, lean proteins, and whole grains, which can help regulate blood sugar levels. High-fibre foods and those low in refined sugars are particularly beneficial.
   o Avoiding Processed Foods: Minimise intake of processed and sugary foods, which can cause rapid blood sugar spikes and exacerbate inflammation. Focus on whole, unprocessed foods instead.
   o Regular Meals: Eating regular, balanced meals helps prevent large fluctuations in blood sugar levels. Aim for consistent mealtimes to maintain stable blood sugar levels.
2. **Reducing Insulin Spikes:**
   o Intermittent Fasting: Implementing intermittent fasting can help manage insulin levels by allowing periods of fasting that reduce insulin secretion and improve insulin sensitivity. This can lower inflammation and promote overall health.
   o Low-Glycaemic Foods: Incorporate foods with a low glycaemic index (GI) to minimise insulin spikes. Low-GI foods release glucose

slowly into the bloodstream, preventing rapid increases in insulin levels.
- ○ Healthy Fats and Proteins: Include healthy fats (such as avocados, nuts, and olive oil) and proteins (such as lean meats and legumes) in your meals to support stable insulin levels and metabolic health.

The Role of Intermittent Fasting in Reducing Inflammation

Intermittent fasting offers several benefits that can help manage inflammation:

- **Improved Insulin Sensitivity**: Intermittent fasting enhances insulin sensitivity and reduces insulin resistance, leading to more stable blood sugar levels and lower inflammation.
- **Enhanced Cellular Repair**: During fasting periods, the body engages in autophagy, a process that removes damaged cells and regenerates new ones. This cellular repair mechanism helps reduce inflammation and supports overall health.
- **Reduction in Inflammatory Markers**: Research indicates that intermittent fasting can lower levels of inflammatory markers, such as C-reactive protein (CRP), which are associated with chronic inflammation and various diseases.
- **Weight Management**: By supporting weight loss and reducing excess body fat, intermittent fasting helps lower chronic inflammation. Maintaining a healthy weight further contributes

to reduced inflammation and improved overall health.

Understanding inflammation and its impact on health is crucial for managing and preventing chronic diseases. By addressing factors such as unstable blood sugar levels and insulin spikes, and incorporating strategies like intermittent fasting, you can effectively reduce inflammation and enhance overall well-being.

Integrating these strategies into your lifestyle can help you achieve a healthier balance and mitigate the risk of inflammation-related conditions. As always, consult with a healthcare professional before making significant changes to your diet or fasting routine, especially if you have pre-existing health conditions. With informed choices and the right approach, you can take control of your health and well-being.

Chapter 7: Lies I Was Told (or Told Myself)

For years, I held on to ideas and advice that only led to frustration and disappointment. These were the "truths" I thought I had to live by—rules I followed strictly, yet never saw the promised results. As I reflect on my journey, I realise that some of the biggest obstacles I faced weren't just physical but mental. These were the lies I was told—or worse, the lies I told myself.

1. "You Have to Eat Less to Lose Weight"

Cutting calories seemed logical, but all it did was leave me hungry, irritable, and discouraged. The idea that starving myself was the only way to slim down was a lie that led to endless cycles of bingeing and guilt.

2. "Breakfast Is the Most Important Meal of the Day"

Every morning, I forced myself to eat, believing it was essential for my metabolism. What I didn't know was that this "must-do" was preventing my body from tapping into its natural fat-burning mode.

3. "Healthy Eating Is All About Low Fat and High Fibre"

I was convinced that low-fat yogurt, wholemeal bread, and high-fibre cereals were the epitome of healthy eating. But these "healthy" choices were packed with hidden sugars, artificial sweeteners, and chemicals designed to make them palatable. Far from nourishing my body, they spiked my blood sugar, increased cravings, and contributed to weight gain. The low-fat yogurt, for instance, was often loaded with more sugar than a chocolate bar, and wholemeal bread, despite its fibre content, was full of refined carbs that offered little nutritional value.

4. "Choose Skimmed Milk or Oat Milk Over Whole Milk"

For years, I believed that opting for skimmed milk or even oat milk was the healthier choice, avoiding the fats in whole milk that I thought were the enemy. But I was wrong. Skimmed milk, stripped of its natural fats, is left with little nutritional value. Worse, it spikes blood sugar levels, leading to insulin surges that leave you hungrier and craving more. Oat milk, which I thought was a wholesome alternative, is often loaded with added sugars and lacks the nutritional density of real milk. By choosing these "healthier" options, I was inadvertently sabotaging my efforts, constantly feeling unsatisfied and wondering why I couldn't control my appetite. It turns out that whole milk, with its natural fats, is far more satiating and supports stable blood sugar levels, which is key to avoiding those mid-morning hunger pangs.

5. "Avoid Eggs, Red Meat, and Fats for a Healthier Heart"

For years, I avoided foods like eggs, red meat, and full-fat dairy, believing they were bad for my heart and waistline. I was told that eggs would raise my cholesterol, red meat would clog my arteries, and fats would make me gain weight. But what I didn't know was that these foods are rich in nutrients essential for optimal health. Eggs provide high-quality protein and vital nutrients, red meat offers iron and B vitamins, and good fats like those in avocados, butter, and olive oil support brain function, hormone production, and energy levels.

One of the biggest lies I fell for was swapping real butter for margarine or spreads made with rapeseed (canola) oil, thinking it was a healthier option. The truth is, margarine and these so-called "heart-healthy" spreads are often loaded with trans fats, synthetic additives, and highly processed oils that can do more harm than good. Unlike these artificial alternatives, grass-fed butter is a natural source of healthy saturated fats, including conjugated linoleic acid (CLA), which has been shown to support weight loss and reduce inflammation. Grass-fed butter is also rich in fat-soluble vitamins like A, D, and K2, which are crucial for bone health, immune function, and cardiovascular health.

However, there is an even larger concern that needs addressing: the increased prescription of statins to lower cholesterol and the widespread adherence to low-fat diets. While these measures have been promoted as solutions for heart health, there is growing evidence suggesting that they may be contributing to a rise in mental health issues and brain diseases, such as Alzheimer's. **Cholesterol is essential for brain function,** as it plays a key role in the structure and function of brain cells. By lowering cholesterol too aggressively, we might be impairing cognitive function and exacerbating neurological conditions. The low-fat rhetoric and the over-prescription of statins may inadvertently be fuelling the reported increase in mental health disorders, further complicating our understanding of diet and health.

By avoiding nutrient-dense foods and replacing them with processed, low-fat alternatives full of sugars and unhealthy oils, I was left unsatisfied, hungrier, and constantly craving the wrong things. The real culprits behind many of the health issues we face aren't natural fats but the processed products that have replaced them in our diets. Switching back to real, wholesome foods like eggs, red meat, and grass-fed butter was a turning point in my journey to better health.

6. "You Need Three Meals a Day for a Balanced Diet"
One of the most deeply ingrained beliefs is that we need to eat three meals a day—breakfast, lunch, and dinner. But what if the problem isn't that we eat too much, but that we eat too often? We've been programmed to believe that constant eating is necessary, but our bodies weren't designed for this. Frequent meals keep our insulin levels high, making it harder to burn stored fat and easier to gain weight. By constantly feeding ourselves, we deny our bodies the chance to tap into their natural energy reserves. Intermittent fasting taught me that it's okay—and often beneficial—not to eat constantly. It's about listening to our bodies and fuelling them when they truly need it, not just because the clock says it's time to eat.

7. "If You Get Sick, There's a Pill for That"
Another lie we've been conditioned to believe is that there's a quick fix for every ailment, often in the form of a pill. When I felt unwell, rarely did a GP ask about my diet or lifestyle. Instead, I was prescribed medications that sometimes alleviated one problem but often caused others. The root cause—what I was or wasn't eating—was almost never addressed. I've

since learned that food can either be our medicine or our poison. Poor dietary choices can lead to a cascade of health issues, while the right foods can heal, restore, and energise. The truth is, many of our chronic health problems stem from what we put on our plates, yet conventional medicine often overlooks this in favour of a pharmaceutical solution. By changing how I eat, I found relief from issues that no prescription ever fully resolved. It turns out that what I needed wasn't more medication—it was a better understanding of how to nourish my body.

8. "Toxic Oils Are in Everything"
One of the biggest shocks for me was discovering the prevalence of toxic oils—like soybean, corn, rapeseed (canola), and sunflower oil—in nearly every processed food. These oils are cheap, but they are also highly processed, unstable, and loaded with unhealthy omega-6 fatty acids. When consumed in excess, they disrupt our body's delicate balance of omega-3 to omega-6 fatty acids, leading to chronic inflammation. But the damage doesn't stop there. These oils can also disrupt our hormones, contributing to weight gain, mood swings, and metabolic issues. They interfere with the body's ability to produce hormones correctly, which can lead to a range of problems from irregular menstrual cycles to increased stress and anxiety. Replacing these toxic oils with healthy fats like olive oil, coconut oil, and butter was a game-changer for me, helping to stabilise my hormones and reduce inflammation.

9. "Exercise More, Eat Less"
I spent hours at the gym, trying to work off the extra weight, but the scale barely moved. The lie that

exercise alone could undo poor eating habits kept me trapped in a cycle of overworking and under-eating.

10. "Being Overweight Is My Fault"
Perhaps the most damaging lie of all was believing that my struggles were due to a lack of willpower. I blamed myself for not trying hard enough when the real issue was that I was misled by faulty advice and misinformation. I wasn't failing because I lacked discipline—I was failing because I was following the wrong guidance.

Now, I understand that the constant cravings and hunger pangs weren't a reflection of my lack of control; they were signals from my brain that it wasn't getting access to the nutrient-dense food it needed to carry out essential processes. My body was starved of the right nutrients, despite being fed regularly. This relentless hunger was exacerbated by the frequent spikes in my blood sugar levels, a result of eating through the day while following the "three meals a day" diatribe. Every time my blood sugar spiked and then crashed, my brain sent out distress signals, making me crave more food—especially sugars and carbs—to quickly restore energy.

What I didn't realise was that this cycle was a recipe for weight gain and poor health, not a sustainable way to live. The traditional advice I was following wasn't just unhelpful; it was actively working against my body's needs. Once I broke free from these misconceptions and started listening to my body, everything changed. The battle wasn't with my willpower—it was with the misinformation that had been guiding my choices.

Discovering the truth behind the lies I had been told—and the ones I told myself—was nothing short of life-changing. For years, I blamed myself for not having enough willpower, for failing at diets, and for feeling constantly hungry and unsatisfied. But now, I see that the problem wasn't me; it was the flawed advice that led me astray. Understanding how my body truly works and what it needs has been incredibly empowering. I'm no longer trapped in a cycle of cravings, hunger, and guilt. Instead, I'm finally living with the energy, health, and confidence I've been chasing for decades.

But this journey isn't just about me. I'm on a mission to share what I've learned with my kids, ensuring they don't fall into the same traps. I want them—and everyone else who will listen—to know that good health isn't about deprivation or willpower; it's about understanding how our bodies function and giving them the right fuel. This truth has set me free, and now, I'm determined to spread the word far and wide.

Chapter 8: My Journey with Intermittent Fasting

Starting the Journey: The First Few Weeks

In my mid-fifties, I was really starting to feel and look my age and after years of grappling with my weight (despite my deep knowledge of nutrition), I faced a growing frustration. My youthful ability to shed pounds quickly through short-term diets had long since faded. The extra two stone I carried became increasingly noticeable and disheartening. Decades of dieting had left me feeling defeated and frustrated, especially after an unsuccessful 'Atkins-style' diet before my wedding in 2002. Though I had managed to lose a few pounds, I never reached my goal weight and felt hungry and deprived throughout the process.

When I discovered intermittent fasting in August 2023, the change was nothing short of transformative. Intrigued by the insights of Davinia Taylor and Dr. Mindy Pelz, I felt a spark of hope for the first time. Their perspectives on how our bodies use energy and how continuous food consumption disrupts our natural balance, was truly refreshing. With the support of my husband, we decided to embark on this new journey, gradually moving to a narrowed eating window from 4pm to 8pm daily. The first few weeks were an adjustment period—managing hunger and learning to eat within a restricted timeframe required patience. However, the steady transition and tricks to reduce the cravings made the adjustment easier, and after 4 or 5 days I noticed improvements in both my energy and mood.

Adjusting to the Fasting Window

As my body adapted to the new fasting routine, I started to experience a sense of control over my eating habits. Structuring my meals to fit within the 4pm to 8pm window became second nature. I focused on making our meals balanced and nutrient-dense, including eggs, good fats, vegetables, lean proteins, whole grains and delicious sour dough bread. Sauerkraut and Kefir (to break my fast) ensured regular consumption of gut friendly bacteria and blueberries with natural Greek yoghurt became a daily staple to that I used to close my eating window, before 8pm each evening. This not only helped in managing hunger but also ensured I was getting the essential nutrients I needed, so my cravings all but disappeared. The changes were gradual but noticeable. I found that my energy levels were more stable, and I felt more focused throughout the day.

Introducing Longer Fasts

Once we felt comfortable with the 4:20 fasting schedule, my husband and I decided to experiment with longer fasting periods. We began incorporating 24-hour fasts and eventually progressed to 36-hour, 48-hour, and even a 72-hour fast! These extended fasts were challenging but incredibly rewarding. They not only accelerated my weight loss but also provided a sense of mental clarity and focus that I hadn't experienced before. The longer fasting periods helped us both to reset and deepen our understanding of how intermittent fasting could be tailored to meet our individual needs. To maintain our energy levels during longer fasts, we made sure to replenish electrolytes with a blend of Celtic salt and lemon juice dissolved in water. Additionally, we found that a teaspoon or two of peanut butter (check that it is free from any 'bad' oils), and "fat-coffees" (black coffee mixed with some grass-fed butter) provided a satisfying energy boost—trust me, it's worth trying! For those seeking convenient alternatives, **Davinia Taylor's WillPowders** line offers MCT Oil, Electrolytes, and Keto Powders that serve a similar purpose; helping to sustain energy and focus during fasting.

These simple interventions—electrolytes, fat-coffees, and MCT oil—are powerful tools that supply your brain the energy it needs while fasting, reducing hunger pangs and cravings. Here's how they work:

1. Electrolytes (Celtic Salt and Lemon Juice):

Electrolytes are essential minerals like sodium, potassium, and magnesium that our bodies need to function properly. When fasting, your body quickly uses up its stored electrolytes, leading to fatigue, headaches, and increased hunger signals. By consuming a blend of Celtic salt and lemon juice in water, you replenish these vital minerals, keeping your energy stable and your brain functioning optimally. This helps prevent the brain from triggering unnecessary hunger signals, as it knows the body's nutrient needs are being met.

2. Fat-Coffees (Black Coffee with Grass-Fed Butter):

Fat-coffees are an excellent way to provide your brain with the fuel it craves during a fast. The healthy fats from grass-fed butter are quickly converted into ketones—a premium energy source that the brain loves. When your brain has access to this steady energy, it doesn't send out panic signals for more food. Instead, it remains calm, reducing cravings and hunger pangs. This makes fasting not only easier but also more sustainable.

3. MCT Oil:
MCT (Medium-Chain Triglyceride) oil is derived from coconut oil and sometimes palm oil and is often found in keto supplements. MCT oil contains concentrated forms of specific fatty acids—mainly caprylic and capric acids—that are easier for the body to convert into energy. Unlike long-chain triglycerides found in most fats, MCTs are rapidly absorbed by the liver, where they are quickly turned into ketones, a powerful fuel source for the brain.

These ketones are immediately available for use by the brain, offering a quick and efficient energy boost. Incorporating MCT oil into your routine can further stabilise your energy levels and keep hunger at bay during fasting. This helps the brain transition smoothly to using stored fat for energy, reducing the need for constant food intake.

Together, these interventions work to provide your brain with the energy it needs, reducing the constant signals that drive hunger and cravings. By calming the brain's response, fasting becomes more manageable, allowing your body to tap into stored fat without the discomfort of constant hunger.

Chapter 9: The Positive Changes We Experienced

Health Improvements: From Snoring to Energy Levels

The health improvements we experienced through intermittent fasting were profound. For my husband, the most noticeable change was the complete elimination of his snoring, which we attributed to better sleep quality and reduced inflammation. I felt a significant boost in my overall energy levels and my aching joints disappeared within a few short weeks. Our enhanced well-being went beyond just weight loss; we both found ourselves more resilient to everyday stresses and less susceptible to common illnesses.

Weight Loss Milestones

The weight loss was one of the most gratifying outcomes of our intermittent fasting journey. This wasn't just a matter of aesthetics; it represented a return to a healthier, more vibrant version of us; my mobility improved, and my ankles didn't swell in the heat or after a long day on my feet. I was thrilled to fit into clothes from my early 20's and felt revitalised in ways I hadn't thought possible. This success was achieved without the hunger and irritability that characterised my past dieting experiences, nor the nagging sense that I'd pile it all back on in a week or two; proving that sustainable health can indeed be simpler than I had imagined.

Emotional and Psychological Benefits

The emotional and psychological benefits of intermittent fasting were as significant as the physical ones. It helped me develop a healthier relationship with food, fostering a more mindful approach to eating. We both experienced reduced 'guilt' around mealtimes and found ourselves more attuned to our bodies' natural hunger cues. The mental clarity (no more brain fog) and improved mood contributed to an overall sense of well-being, reinforcing the idea that intermittent fasting was not just a diet but a holistic approach to improved health.

Another hidden benefit of Intermittent Fasting

By adopting intermittent fasting and essentially eating just one meal a day, we significantly reduced our weekly food intake. Instead of the typical 21 meals per week, (28 if you count one daily snack), we cut down to just 7, and sometimes even fewer if we were doing a longer fast. It goes without saying that this shift obviously **had a profound and positive impact on our food budget.**

With fewer meals to prepare, we invested in higher-quality ingredients without increasing our spending. By focusing on quality over quantity, we were able to purchase organic produce, grass-fed meats, and other nutrient-dense foods that truly nourish the body. This approach not only enhanced the taste and enjoyment of our meals but also ensured that each meal provided maximum nutritional value.

Reducing the number of meals meant less time spent on meal prep and grocery shopping, allowing us to focus more on savouring each meal and enjoying the benefits of better health. Plus, the savings on our food budget provided the flexibility to indulge in premium ingredients that support our overall well-being, making this lifestyle both sustainable and satisfying.

Chapter 10: How We Made It Work

Transitioning Gradually: A Practical Guide

Our journey with intermittent fasting began with a gradual transition, which was crucial for our success. Starting with a manageable eating window and slowly incorporating longer fasts helped our bodies adapt without overwhelming us. I recommend starting with a 12-hour fasting period and gradually extending it as you become more comfortable. We began by pushing our first meal back by 45 mins for the first week, and then further back by an hour for the following weeks until we got to 4pm. At the same time, we introduced the 'no-food past 8pm' rule.

Managing Cravings and Hunger

Managing cravings and hunger was a significant part of our intermittent fasting journey. Staying hydrated with water, black coffee, herbal teas, and electrolyte-rich drinks helped curb hunger and maintain energy levels. We also learned to distract ourselves with activities and focus on the benefits of fasting rather than the temporary discomfort. Planning balanced meals that included plenty of fibre, protein, and healthy fats helped keep us satisfied during eating windows.

Tips for Staying Hydrated and Energised

Staying hydrated and energised during fasting periods is essential. We made it a habit to drink plenty of water throughout the day and incorporated hydrating foods like cucumbers and leafy greens into our meals. Adding a pinch of salt and lemon to our water or consuming electrolyte supplements also helped maintain our energy levels.

Chapter 11: Fasting Variations and Adaptations

Different Fasting Protocols

Dr. Mindy Pelz is a renowned expert in the field of health and wellness, celebrated for her extensive research and advocacy on the benefits of fasting. As a functional medicine practitioner, she has dedicated her career to exploring and promoting the transformative effects of fasting on the body and mind. With a focus on personalised health strategies, Dr. Pelz combines cutting-edge scientific insights with practical advice to help individuals optimise their well-being. Her work emphasises how different fasting protocols can enhance overall health, support metabolic function, and contribute to long-term wellness. I discovered Dr. Mindy through her book **'Fast Like a Girl'** and then her You Tube Channel, where she has over 1.2 million followers. Dr. Pelz empowers people to take control of their health by understanding and applying the principles of fasting in their daily lives.

Below is a summary of the benefits of different fasting lengths according to Dr. Mindy Pelz:

13-15 Hour Fast (Circadian Rhythm Fast)
Benefits: This is the easiest and most sustainable fasting window and aligns with the body's natural circadian rhythm. It helps to stabilise blood sugar, initiate fat burning, and regulate insulin levels. This type of fast also supports gut health by giving the

digestive system a break and improving sleep quality.

Who it's for: Beginners and those looking to maintain general health.

16-18 Hour Fast (Intermittent Fasting)

Benefits: Extending the fast to 16-18 hours boosts fat burning and increases human growth hormone (HGH) levels, which supports muscle growth and fat loss. This fasting window also promotes autophagy, a process where the body cleans out damaged cells and regenerates new ones, enhancing cellular repair.

Who it's for: Those aiming for weight loss, improved metabolic health, and anti-aging benefits.

24-Hour Fast (One Meal a Day - OMAD)

Benefits: A 24-hour fast allows for a deeper level of autophagy, providing significant cellular repair. This length of fasting helps reset the gut, improves mental clarity, and can lower inflammation. Additionally, it can help break through weight loss plateaus by pushing the body into ketosis, a state where fat is used as the primary energy source.

Who it's for: Intermediate fasters who want to improve mental focus, reduce inflammation, and boost metabolism.

36-Hour Fast

Benefits: A 36-hour fast further enhances autophagy and fat burning. This fasting length is effective for resetting insulin sensitivity, which is particularly beneficial for those with metabolic syndrome or type 2 diabetes. It also promotes a deep state of ketosis, providing mental clarity and sustained energy levels.

Who it's for: Advanced fasters who want to reset their metabolism, improve insulin sensitivity, and reduce chronic inflammation.

48-Hour Fast

Benefits: A 48-hour fast takes autophagy and cellular repair to a profound level. This fasting length significantly lowers inflammation, enhances detoxification processes, and deeply resets the immune system. It's also beneficial for those seeking to reverse chronic conditions, as it can dramatically improve metabolic health and insulin sensitivity.

Who it's for: Experienced fasters looking for a comprehensive reset, especially those managing chronic health issues or seeking advanced autophagy benefits.

72-Hour Fast

Benefits: The 72-hour fast is often referred to as the ultimate fasting reset. It completely rejuvenates the immune system by stimulating the production of new white blood cells. This fast is highly effective for reducing inflammation, enhancing cognitive function, and improving longevity. It is also a powerful tool for those seeking to reset their health at a deep cellular level.

Who it's for: Advanced fasters who are looking for a complete health reset or who are preparing for or recovering from significant health challenges.

Varying the lengths of your fasts can maximise health benefits by tapping into different physiological processes. Shorter fasts are great for daily maintenance, while longer fasts can be used periodically for deeper healing and metabolic resets. It's important to listen to your body and progress gradually, especially if you are new to fasting.

Adapting Fasting for Different Lifestyles and Needs

Fasting is a versatile and powerful tool for improving health, but it's not a one-size-fits-all approach. Different lifestyles, individual needs, and health conditions can all influence the best way to incorporate fasting into your routine. Whether you're a busy professional, an athlete, a parent, or someone with specific health goals, fasting can be tailored to fit your unique situation. Here's how to adapt fasting to different lifestyles and needs for maximum benefits.

1. For Busy Professionals

If you have a demanding career with long hours and little flexibility, fasting can still be a valuable part of your health routine. Intermittent fasting with a 16:8 or 18:6 window is often the easiest to incorporate. You can skip breakfast and eat within an 8-hour window, such as from 12 PM to 8 PM, aligning your meals with your work schedule.

Tips:
- Plan meals ahead of time to avoid unhealthy, last-minute food choices.
- Use coffee or herbal teas to help manage hunger during the fasting window.

- Focus on nutrient-dense meals to sustain energy throughout the day.

2. For Athletes and Highly Active Individuals
Athletes and those with active lifestyles need to ensure they're getting enough nutrients to fuel their workouts and recovery. For this group, fasting can be integrated with careful attention to nutrient timing, particularly around workouts.
   Tips:
   - Time your eating window to coincide with your workout for optimal energy and recovery.
   - Include plenty of protein and complex carbohydrates in your meals to support muscle repair and glycogen replenishment.
   - Consider shorter fasting windows or occasional extended fasts on rest days.

3. For Parents and Caregivers
Managing a household and caring for others can make sticking to a strict fasting schedule challenging. Flexibility is key for parents, who may benefit from shorter, more manageable fasting windows, such as 12:12 or 14:10.
   Tips:
   - Involve the family in healthy eating habits to make meal planning easier.
   - Use shorter fasting windows that fit around family meals.
   - Prioritise quality over quantity; focus on whole foods and balanced meals when you do eat.

4. For Those with a Menstrual Cycle
Hormonal fluctuations throughout the menstrual cycle can impact energy levels, appetite, and how the body

responds to fasting. It's important to adapt fasting protocols according to these cycles.

Tips:
- During the follicular phase (after menstruation), the body may be more resilient to longer fasts, making it an ideal time to try 16:8 or 18:6 fasting windows.
- During the luteal phase (after ovulation), shorter fasting windows (12:12 or 14:10) might be more suitable to accommodate increased energy needs and cravings.
- Consider incorporating nutrient-dense, hormone-supportive foods like leafy greens, healthy fats, and complex carbs to support your cycle.

5. For Those with Chronic Health Conditions

If you have a chronic health condition such as diabetes, thyroid issues, or an autoimmune disorder, fasting can still be beneficial, but it must be approached with caution and tailored to your specific needs.

Tips:
- Consult with a healthcare provider before starting any fasting regimen, especially if you are on medication.
- Start with shorter fasts (12:12) and gradually increase the duration as tolerated.
- Monitor your symptoms closely and adjust as needed to ensure that fasting supports, rather than aggravates, your condition.

6. For Older Adults

As we age, maintaining muscle mass, bone health, and overall energy becomes increasingly important. Older adults can still benefit from fasting, but it's essential to prioritise nutrition and not overly restrict caloric intake.

Tips:
- Use shorter fasting windows to ensure adequate nutrient intake.
- Focus on protein-rich meals to support muscle maintenance and bone health.
- Incorporate regular physical activity, including strength training, to complement fasting.

7. For Those Seeking Weight Loss

If weight loss is your primary goal, fasting can be a highly effective strategy, especially when combined with mindful eating and regular exercise. Varying fasting lengths and incorporating longer fasts (24-hour, 36-hour, or 48-hour fasts) can help overcome plateaus and accelerate fat loss.

Tips:
- Start with intermittent fasting (16:8) and progress to longer fasts as your body adapts.
- Avoid breaking your fast with high-calorie, low-nutrient foods; focus on balanced, whole-food meals.
- Combine fasting with resistance training to preserve muscle mass while losing fat.

The beauty of fasting lies in its flexibility. By adapting your fasting approach to fit your lifestyle, activity level, and specific health needs, you can reap the benefits without feeling restricted or overwhelmed. Remember, **the best fasting plan is one that you can maintain comfortably over the long term**. Listen to your body, be patient with yourself, and embrace fasting as a versatile tool to enhance your health and well-being.

Chapter 12: Tips for Successful Fasting

Identifying Your Fasting Style: 16:8 and Beyond

Finding the right fasting style is essential for long-term success. We initially started with the 16:8 method, where we fasted for 16 hours and ate within an 8-hour window, but quickly moved to 20:4 or an OMAD (one meal a day) style of eating. However, Dr. Mindy Pelz's approach to fasting provided us with additional strategies that enhanced our experience.

We experimented with different fasting durations, such as 24-hour fasts, and explored longer fasting periods, including 36-hour and 48-hour fasts. This flexibility allowed us to find what worked best for our bodies and lifestyle. The key is to start with a method that aligns with your personal routine and gradually explore other fasting styles as you become more comfortable.

Tricks to Keep Cravings at Bay During Intermittent Fasting

1. **Bulletproof Coffee**
   - This high-fat coffee blend made with butter and MCT oil can help keep you full and provide sustained energy during fasting periods. The fat content can also help manage hunger pangs.
2. **Butter in Coffee**
   - Adding a small amount of unsalted butter to your coffee can provide a creamy texture and help

keep you satiated. This approach can also offer a boost of energy and help reduce cravings.

3. **Electrolytes**
   - Electrolyte Supplements: Use supplements containing sodium, potassium, and magnesium to maintain electrolyte balance, especially during longer fasts or if you're sweating more than usual. Ensure they are free of sugars or artificial sweeteners.
   - Salt: A pinch of sea salt or Himalayan salt in your water can help replenish electrolytes and maintain balance during fasting periods.

4. **Hydration**
   - Water: Drinking plenty of water is essential to stay hydrated and can help reduce hunger pangs.
   - Herbal Teas: Non-caloric herbal teas like peppermint, chamomile, or ginger can aid in hydration and offer a comforting ritual during fasting.

5. **Black Coffee**
   - Plain black coffee can help suppress appetite and provide a caffeine boost without breaking your fast, also enhancing mental clarity.

6. **Green Tea**
   - Contains catechins that may help with appetite suppression and provides a mild caffeine boost.

7. **Bone Broth**
   - Rich in minerals and electrolytes, bone broth can help stave off hunger and support electrolyte balance. Ensure it's free of added sugars or high-calorie ingredients.

8. **Fibre Supplements**
   - Psyllium Husk: Adding this to water may help with feelings of fullness due to its high fibre

content. Remember to drink plenty of water with it.

9. **Apple Cider Vinegar**
    o A small amount (1-2 tablespoons) diluted in water before or during fasting may aid in appetite control and digestion.

10. **Mint or Gum**
    o Chewing gum or sucking on a mint can help manage cravings and freshen breath but be cautious with gum if it contains sugar or artificial sweeteners.

11. **Adaptogens**
    o Adaptogenic Herbs: Herbs like ashwagandha or rhodiola can help manage stress and cortisol levels, potentially reducing cravings.

12. **Mindful Eating**
    o Mindful Practices: Engage in mindfulness or meditation to manage emotional eating and stress-related cravings. Techniques like deep breathing or guided meditation can also help.

13. **Balanced Meals**
    o Nutrient-Dense Meals: Focus on meals high in protein, healthy fats, and fibre when you eat to keep you full longer and reduce cravings.

14. **Sleep and Stress Management**
    o Quality Sleep: Ensure adequate, restful sleep to help control hunger and cravings.
    o Stress Management: Use techniques such as yoga, journaling, or breathing exercises to manage stress and prevent stress-related overeating.

Incorporating these strategies can help make intermittent fasting more manageable and effective. Listen to your body and adjust as needed to maintain both physical and mental well-being during your fasting periods.

Overcoming Plateaus

Experiencing a weight loss plateau is a common and sometimes frustrating aspect of any weight loss programme including intermittent fasting. A plateau occurs when progress stalls despite sticking to your routine. However, understanding how to navigate and overcome these plateaus can help you continue making progress. Here are strategies and insights to help you push through these challenging periods.

Understanding Weight Loss Plateaus

Weight loss plateaus happen when your body adapts to a new routine or weight loss slows down after an initial period of success. During a plateau, the body's metabolism may adjust to the reduced caloric intake or changes in diet and exercise, making it harder to continue losing weight at the same rate.

Strategies for Overcoming Plateaus

1. **Reassess Your Fasting Routine:**
   o Evaluate Your Fasting Schedule: Take a closer look at your current fasting schedule. If you've been following the same pattern for a while, your body might have adapted. Consider making changes to your fasting window or the frequency of your fasting days. For example, if you've been on a 16:8 schedule, try adjusting to a 20:4 or 14:10 schedule for a few weeks.
   o Incorporate Periodic Extended Fasts: As advised by Dr. Mindy Pelz, adding occasional extended fasts (such as 24, 36, or even 48 hours) can help overcome plateaus. These extended fasts can help reset your

metabolism and provide a new stimulus for fat loss. Plan these extended fasts carefully and ensure you are well-hydrated and prepared before starting.

2. **Adjust Your Eating Window:**
   - Alternate Fasting Periods: Try alternating between shorter and longer fasting periods. For example, if you normally fast for 16 hours, experiment with a 24-hour fast once a week or switch to a 12-hour eating window on some days. This variation can prevent your body from adapting to a single routine and stimulate continued progress.
   - Re-evaluate Meal Timing: The timing of your meals can impact your progress. If you've been eating at the same times every day, try shifting your eating window earlier or later to see if it affects your results.

3. **Modify Your Diet:**
   - Examine Your Food Choices: Ensure that your meals are balanced and nutrient dense. Sometimes, plateaus occur due to changes in dietary habits, such as increased consumption of processed foods or hidden sugars. Pay special attention to your fruit intake—**while fruits are nutritious, they can be high in natural sugars**. Opt for lower-sugar fruits like berries and consume them in moderation. Additionally, focus on whole foods, high in fibre and protein, and low in refined carbohydrates. Avoid excessive snacking or consuming high-calorie foods that may hinder your progress.

- Track Your Intake: Keep a food diary or use a nutrition app to track what you're eating. This can help identify any hidden calories or dietary patterns that might be affecting your progress.

4. **Increase Physical Activity:**
   - Incorporate New Exercises: If you've been doing the same exercise routine, your body may have adapted, leading to a plateau. Introduce new workouts or increase the intensity of your current routine. For example, add strength training if you've been focusing on cardio, or try high-intensity interval training (HIIT) to boost your metabolism.
   - Vary Exercise Types: Mixing up different types of physical activity can prevent adaptation and stimulate different muscle groups. Consider activities like swimming, cycling, or yoga to complement your regular workouts.

5. **Evaluate Your Sleep and Stress Levels:**
   - Improve Sleep Quality: Inadequate sleep can hinder weight loss progress and contribute to plateaus. Aim for 7-9 hours of quality sleep per night and establish a consistent sleep routine. Avoid screens before bedtime and create a relaxing environment.
   - Manage Stress: Chronic stress can affect hormonal balance and lead to weight loss plateaus. Implement stress-reduction techniques such as meditation, deep breathing exercises, or hobbies you enjoy.

6. **Stay Hydrated:**

- Monitor Fluid Intake: Proper hydration is crucial for overall health and can impact weight loss. Ensure you're drinking enough water throughout the day. Sometimes, plateaus can be attributed to fluid retention or dehydration.

7. **Seek Professional Advice:**
   - Consult with a Specialist: If you continue to experience a plateau despite adjusting, consider consulting a healthcare professional or a registered dietitian. They can provide personalised advice and help identify any underlying issues that might be affecting your progress.

Examples of Applying These Strategies

1. *Weekly Variation*: If you normally fast for 16 hours daily, try extending your fast to 24 hours once a week. This change can help reset your metabolism and potentially jumpstart your progress.
2. *Dietary Adjustment*: If you've been consuming more snacks or processed foods, focus on clean eating by preparing meals with whole, unprocessed ingredients. For instance, replace sugary snacks with nuts and seeds or a bowl of natural Greek yoghurt and blueberries.
3. *Exercise Routine*: If you've been walking daily, add strength training exercises twice a week to build muscle and boost metabolism. Incorporate activities like weightlifting, resistance bands, or bodyweight exercises.
4. *Stress Management*: If stress has been a factor, incorporate mindfulness practices into your routine. Set aside 10-15 minutes daily for meditation or deep breathing exercises.

Weight loss plateaus are a common part of the intermittent fasting journey, but they can be managed with a strategic approach. By reassessing your fasting routine, adjusting your diet, increasing physical activity, and addressing factors like sleep and stress, you can overcome plateaus and continue making progress. Remember, persistence and flexibility are key. With thoughtful adjustments and a proactive mindset, you can navigate plateaus and achieve your health goals.

Social and Family Life: How to Fast in a Busy World

Integrating intermittent fasting into a busy lifestyle and social life can indeed present challenges, but with some planning, flexibility, and communication, it can be seamlessly incorporated into daily routines. Here's a more detailed look at how to manage fasting amidst the demands of family life and social commitments.

Communication is Key
One of the most effective strategies for maintaining your fasting routine while navigating social situations is open communication. Letting family and friends know about your fasting schedule helps manage expectations and reduce potential misunderstandings. Here are some practical steps:

- **Informing Family and Friends**: Share your fasting plan with close family members and friends. Explain why you're adopting this approach and how it benefits you. Most people will understand and support your decision once they know it's important to you.

- **Discussing Social Events**: Before attending social gatherings, communicate your fasting schedule to the host. You can discuss possible timing adjustments or let them know you may bring a small meal or snack that aligns with your eating window.
- **Setting Boundaries**: Politely set boundaries regarding mealtimes and food offerings. For instance, if a gathering involves a meal outside your eating window, let the host know in advance that you'll eat before or after the event.

Planning and Preparation

Effective planning can make it easier to stick to your fasting routine without feeling deprived or isolated. Here are some tips for integrating fasting into your busy lifestyle:

- **Meal Prep**: Preparing meals in advance can save time and ensure that you have nutritious options available within your eating window. Batch cooking and meal prepping allow you to enjoy home-cooked, healthy meals even on the busiest days.
- **Healthy Snacks**: Keep healthy snacks on hand for when you break your fast. These can include fruits, nuts, yogurt, or protein bars. Having these available ensures that you stay on track without feeling tempted to deviate from your plan.
- **Scheduling Meals**: Coordinate your fasting schedule with your daily activities and appointments. For instance, if you have a meeting or workout session, plan your meals around these events to avoid conflicts.

- **Adaptable Eating Windows**: While it's essential to stick to a routine, being flexible with your eating window, when necessary, can help you manage social commitments better. If a special occasion falls outside your usual eating window, consider adjusting it slightly to accommodate the event without derailing your progress.

Navigating Social Gatherings

Social events and family gatherings can be enjoyable and stress-free while maintaining your fasting routine with these strategies:

- **Planning Your Attendance**: Decide whether to attend social events during your fasting or eating window. If the event falls outside your eating window, consider arriving just before your fast ends or planning to eat beforehand.
- **Bringing Your Own Food**: If you're concerned about food options at social events, bring your own meal or snack that fits within your fasting routine. This can also serve as a conversation starter and helps ensure you have something you can enjoy.
- **Engaging in Social Activities**: Focus on the social aspects of gatherings rather than just the food. Engage in conversations, participate in activities, and enjoy the company of others. This approach helps shift the focus away from eating and keeps the event enjoyable.
- **Adapting to Situations**: If you find yourself in a situation where you need to break your fast, do so mindfully and plan your next fasting window accordingly. Flexibility is key to maintaining balance without compromising your health goals.

- **Exploring Alternative Activities**: Suggest activities that don't revolve around food, such as hiking, games, or cultural events. This helps create social opportunities that align with your fasting routine and provides alternative ways to connect with others.

Examples of Balancing Fasting with Social Life
1. **Family Dinner**: If your family dinner time is outside your eating window, plan to have a small meal before joining the family table. This allows you to participate in the meal without disrupting your fasting routine.
2. **Work Events**: For work-related events that involve meals or snacks, check the event details beforehand and plan your meals around the event. You might choose to eat earlier in the day and attend the event for networking or socialising or bring a healthy snack to enjoy during a break.
3. **Holiday Gatherings**: During holidays or special occasions, where meals are often served outside typical eating windows, adjust your fasting schedule slightly to accommodate the festivities. For instance, extend your eating window on special days and resume your regular schedule the following day.
4. **Weekend Outings**: If you have a day trip or outing planned, prepare portable meals or snacks that fit within your fasting routine. Carry a cooler with pre-prepared options to ensure you stay on track while enjoying your outing.

Balancing intermittent fasting with a busy lifestyle and social commitments requires thoughtful planning and adaptability. By communicating your needs, preparing in advance, and being flexible with your schedule, you can successfully integrate fasting into your daily routine without feeling isolated or deprived. Remember that with the right strategies, fasting can enhance your health and well-being while still allowing you to enjoy social interactions and family life.

Chapter 13: What We Eat During Our Eating Window

Foods to Prioritise: Nutrient-Dense

1. Lean Proteins

High-quality proteins are essential for muscle maintenance, satiety, and overall health. They help stabilise blood sugar levels and keep you full longer.

- **Chicken breast** (organic, free-range if possible)
- **Beef**
- **Turkey**
- **Salmon, mackerel, and sardines** (rich in omega-3 fatty acids)
- **Eggs** (organic, pasture-raised)
- **Greek yogurt** (unsweetened)
- **Tofu and tempeh** (organic, non-GMO)

2. Healthy Fats

Incorporating healthy fats is crucial for brain function, hormone production, and satiety. They help you stay full and provide long-lasting energy.

- **Avocados**
- **Nuts and seeds** (e.g., pistachios, cashew nuts, almonds, walnuts, chia seeds, flaxseeds)
- **Olive oil** (extra virgin)
- **Coconut oil** (cold-pressed, virgin)
- **Grass-fed Butter**
- **Nut butters** (almond, cashew, or peanut, without added sugars or oils)
- **Fatty fish** (salmon, sardines, mackerel)

3. Complex Carbohydrates

Complex carbs provide steady energy and are packed with fibre, vitamins, and minerals. They are essential for breaking your fast with nutrient-dense foods.

- **Sour Dough Bread**
- **Quinoa**
- **Sweet potatoes**
- **Brown rice**
- **Oats** (steel-cut or rolled)
- **Lentils and beans** (black beans, chickpeas, lentils)
- **Whole-grain bread and pasta**

4. Leafy Greens and Vegetables

These are low in calories but high in fibre, vitamins, minerals, and antioxidants. They are excellent for maintaining a balanced diet and supporting overall health.

- **Spinach**
- **Kale**
- **Broccoli**
- **Cauliflower**
- **Brussels sprouts**
- **Courgette**
- **Asparagus**

5. Berries and Low-Sugar Fruits

Berries are rich in antioxidants, fibre, and vitamins, making them an excellent choice for nutrient density without the sugar spike.

- **Blueberries**
- **Strawberries**
- **Raspberries**
- **Blackberries**
- **Apples** (with the skin)
- **Pears** (with the skin)
- **Citrus fruits** (oranges, grapefruits, lemons)

6. Fermented Foods

Fermented foods support gut health, which is critical for digestion, immunity, and overall wellness.

- **Kimchi**
- **Sauerkraut**

- **Kombucha** (low sugar)
- **Kefir** (unsweetened)
- **Miso**
- **Pickles** (fermented, not pickled in vinegar)

7. Bone Broth and Soups

Bone broth is rich in collagen, gelatine, and minerals, making it an excellent way to break a fast gently while providing essential nutrients.

- **Chicken bone broth**
- **Beef bone broth**
- **Vegetable soups** (homemade, with minimal added salt)
- **Miso soup**

8. Herbs and Spices

These add flavour and contain anti-inflammatory and antioxidant properties, helping to enhance the nutritional value of your meals.

- **Turmeric**
- **Ginger**
- **Garlic**
- **Cinnamon**
- **Pepper**
- **Basil, oregano, and thyme**

9. Hydrating Foods

Incorporating foods with high water content helps keep you hydrated and supports overall digestion.

- **Cucumbers**
- **Celery**
- **Watermelon**
- **Lettuce**
- **Tomatoes**

10. Beverages

Staying hydrated is key to successful intermittent fasting. Certain beverages can also support health without breaking your fast.

- **Water** (plain or infused with lemon or cucumber)
- **Herbal teas** (peppermint, chamomile, ginger)
- **Black coffee** (no sugar or cream)
- **Green tea** (rich in antioxidants)

Incorporating these nutritious foods into your eating window will not only help you achieve your weight loss goals but also support your overall health and well-being during your intermittent fasting journey.

Foods to Avoid

To maximise the benefits of intermittent fasting, it's important to avoid or limit certain foods that can sabotage your progress:
- **Refined sugars and sweeteners** (e.g., sodas, candies, pastries)
- **Ultra-processed foods** (e.g., fast food, packaged snacks)
- **Refined grains** (e.g., white bread, white rice, pasta)
- **Trans fats** (e.g., margarine, certain fried foods, many baked goods)
- **Artificial sweeteners and additives** (e.g., aspartame, MSG)
- **Alcohol** (in excess, as it can disrupt metabolism and sleep)

Ultra Processed Foods: What to Look Out For

Processed foods are often laden with ingredients that can undermine your health and weight loss efforts. Understanding what to look for on ingredient labels can help you make informed choices and avoid hidden dangers. Below is a guide to help you navigate the world of processed foods, including a list of harmful additives, chemicals, and sugars that should be avoided.

1. Understand What "Processed" Means

Processed foods are those that have been altered from their natural state for convenience, shelf life, or taste. They often contain unhealthy additives, preservatives, and sugars that contribute to weight gain, inflammation, and chronic health issues.

Common Examples of Processed Foods:

- Sugary cereals
- Packaged snacks (chips, cookies, crackers)
- Instant noodles and soups
- Frozen meals and pizzas
- Canned foods with added salts or sugars
- Sugary beverages, including sodas and fruit juices

2. Check the Ingredient List

Reading the ingredient list is key to identifying processed foods. Avoid products with long ingredient lists, especially those containing artificial additives, preservatives, and hidden sugars.

Key Ingredients to Avoid:

a. Harmful Additives and Chemicals

- **Artificial colours**: Red 40, Yellow 5, Blue 1
- **Artificial Flavors**: Often listed as "flavour" or "artificial flavour"
- **Preservatives**: BHT (Butylated Hydroxytoluene), BHA (Butylated Hydroxyanisole), Sodium benzoate, Potassium sorbate

- **Emulsifiers and thickeners**: Carrageenan, Polysorbate 80, Soy lecithin, Mono- and diglycerides
- **Artificial sweeteners**: Aspartame, Sucralose, Acesulfame K, Saccharin
- **Trans fats**: Partially hydrogenated oils (found in some margarine, baked goods, and fried foods)
- **Flavour enhancers**: Monosodium glutamate (MSG), Disodium inosinate, Disodium guanylate
- **High sodium ingredients**: Sodium nitrite, Sodium phosphate

b. Hidden Sugars and Sweeteners Sugars are often disguised under different names, making it easy to overlook them on labels. Here are some common names for sugars and sweeteners that should be avoided:

- **Common Sugars**:
  - High-fructose corn syrup (HFCS)
  - Corn syrup, corn syrup solids
  - Dextrose
  - Fructose
  - Glucose
  - Maltose
  - Sucrose
  - Cane sugar, cane juice
  - Beet sugar
  - Maltodextrin
- **Natural Sugars (to consume sparingly)**:
  - Agave nectar
  - Honey
  - Maple syrup
  - Coconut sugar
- **Artificial and Low-Calorie Sweeteners**:
  - Aspartame

- Sucralose
- Saccharin
- Acesulfame K
- Neotame

3. Beware of Health Halos

Some processed foods are marketed as "healthy" but can still contain harmful ingredients. Labels like "low-fat," "gluten-free," or "natural" don't necessarily mean the product is good for you. Always read the ingredient list to check for hidden sugars, unhealthy fats, and additives.

4. Focus on Whole, Minimally Processed Foods

Instead of relying on processed options, aim to fill your diet with whole, nutrient-dense foods that are close to their natural state. These foods provide essential nutrients without the unhealthy extras found in processed items.

Whole Foods to Focus On:
- Fresh fruits and vegetables
- Whole grains like quinoa, brown rice, and oats
- Lean proteins such as chicken, fish, and eggs
- Legumes like lentils, beans, and chickpeas
- Healthy fats from nuts, seeds, avocados, and olive oil

5. Meal Prep and Planning

One of the best ways to avoid processed foods is by planning and preparing your meals in advance. This allows you to control the ingredients and avoid the convenience of packaged, processed options.

Meal Prep Tips:
- Cook large portions of grains, proteins, and vegetables for use throughout the week.

- Keep healthy snacks like cut-up veggies, nuts, and berries readily available.
- Prepare sauces, dressings, and marinades at home to avoid store-bought versions loaded with sugars and preservatives.

6. Shop the Perimeter of the Grocery Store
When shopping, stick to the perimeter where fresh produce, meats, and whole grains are usually found. Avoid the inner aisles where most processed and packaged foods are located. If you do venture into these aisles, be selective and stick to your list.

Avoiding processed foods is essential for achieving and maintaining good health. By being vigilant about reading ingredient labels and focusing on whole, unprocessed foods, you can avoid the pitfalls of hidden sugars, harmful additives, and unhealthy fats.

Supplementing for Optimal Health

While many people believe that a well-balanced diet alone should provide all the necessary nutrients for optimal health, the reality is challenging due to various factors. Food quality often varies significantly, and in many cases, the nutritional value of fruits, vegetables, and other staples may be compromised by factors such as soil depletion, pesticides, and storage conditions. Additionally, the actual nutrient content of food can be inconsistent and sometimes unknown. For these reasons, even those who strive to eat healthily may not always meet their nutritional needs solely through diet. In such cases, carefully chosen supplements can play a vital role in filling potential gaps, ensuring that individuals receive adequate levels of essential vitamins and minerals to support overall health and wellness.

On top of a daily multi-vitamin and mineral supplement, as well as high doses vitamin C, this is what I have been taking whilst on my wellness journey.

1. **Essential Supplements**
   - **Omega-3 Fatty Acids**
     - Benefits: Supports heart health, reduces inflammation.
     - Sources: Fish oil supplements or algae-based omega-3 supplements for vegetarians.
   - **Vitamin D**
     - Benefits: Supports bone health, enhances mood.
     - Sources: Vitamin D3 supplements, especially if you have limited sun exposure.
   - **Magnesium**
     - Benefits: Supports muscle and nerve function, helps with sleep.
     - Sources: Magnesium supplements or sprays, or dietary sources like nuts, seeds, and leafy greens.
2. **Gut Health Supplements**
   - **Probiotics**
     - Benefits: Promotes a healthy gut microbiome, aids digestion.
     - Sources: Probiotic supplements or fermented foods like kefir and sauerkraut.
   - **Digestive Enzymes**
     - Benefits: Supports digestion and nutrient absorption.

- Sources: Digestive enzyme supplements, or foods rich in natural enzymes like pineapple and papaya.

3. **Hydration and Electrolytes**
   - **Electrolyte Supplements**
     - Benefits: Helps maintain fluid balance, supports muscle function.
     - Sources: Electrolyte powders or capsules, especially useful during fasting periods.
   - **Hydration Tips**
     - Aim to drink at least 8 glasses of water daily. Incorporate herbal teas and infuse water with fruits for variety.

Chapter 14: The Science Behind Cravings and Nutrition

Understanding the science behind cravings and nutrition is crucial for making informed decisions that support your health goals. Our bodies and brains are wired to crave certain foods, often those high in sugar, salt, and fat. However, by comprehending the underlying reasons for these cravings and how to balance our nutritional intake—especially during fasting—we can make choices that nourish us and help us stay on track.

Why We Crave Certain Foods

Cravings are complex phenomena driven by a combination of biological, psychological, and environmental factors. At their core, cravings are your body's way of signalling a need, whether it's energy, nutrients, or even emotional comfort. Here are some key reasons why we crave certain foods:

1. **Biological Mechanisms**: Our brains are hardwired to seek out high-calorie foods—those rich in sugar and fat—because, historically, these foods were scarce and provided the energy needed for survival. When you consume sugary or fatty foods, your brain releases dopamine, a neurotransmitter associated with pleasure and reward. This creates a reinforcing loop that makes you want to eat those foods again and again.
2. **Nutrient Deficiencies**: Sometimes cravings are your body's way of signalling a nutrient deficiency. For instance, a craving for chocolate might indicate a need for

magnesium, or a craving for salty foods could suggest an imbalance in electrolytes. However, these signals can be misinterpreted, leading us to reach for unhealthy options instead of the nutrient-dense foods our bodies need.

3. **Emotional Triggers**: Stress, boredom, sadness, or even happiness can trigger cravings as we seek comfort in food. I realise now that I spent much of my adult life 'eating my feelings'. Emotional eating often leads to the consumption of high-calorie, low-nutrient foods, which can derail health goals and contribute to weight gain.

4. **Environmental Cues**: Marketing, social situations, and even the sight or smell of food can trigger cravings. Fast food advertisements, for example, are designed to make you crave what they're selling, even if you're not hungry.

The Importance of Nutrient-Rich Eating

One of the most effective ways to combat cravings and support overall health is to prioritise nutrient-rich eating. When your body receives the vitamins, minerals, and macronutrients it needs, cravings for unhealthy foods tend to diminish. Here's why nutrient-dense foods are vital:

1. **Balanced Blood Sugar Levels**: Eating a diet rich in whole foods—like vegetables, fruits, lean proteins, and healthy fats—helps maintain stable blood sugar levels. This stability reduces the spikes and crashes that often lead to cravings for sugary or carb-heavy foods.

2. **Satiety and Satisfaction**: Nutrient-rich foods are often more filling and satisfying because they contain fibre, healthy fats, and protein. These nutrients signal to your brain that you're

full, reducing the likelihood of overeating or reaching for unhealthy snacks.

3. **Support for Metabolic Health**: A diet rich in essential nutrients supports optimal metabolic function, helping your body efficiently convert food into energy, repair cells, and maintain hormonal balance. This reduces the likelihood of craving quick-fix energy sources like sugar.

4. **Mood Regulation**: Nutrient-dense foods, particularly those high in omega-3 fatty acids, B vitamins, and magnesium, play a critical role in mood regulation. A stable mood decreases emotional eating, reducing the risk of cravings triggered by stress or anxiety.

How to Balance Macronutrients During Fasting

Fasting can be a powerful tool for health and weight loss, but it's important to balance your macronutrient intake when you do eat. Proper macronutrient balance ensures that your body gets the energy and nutrients it needs, supports satiety, and prevents cravings. Here's how to approach it:

1. **Prioritise Protein**: Protein is essential for muscle repair, immune function, and overall health. It also has the highest satiety factor among macronutrients, helping you feel full longer. During your eating window, include high-quality protein sources such as eggs, lean meats, fish, legumes, and plant-based options like tofu or tempeh.

2. **Incorporate Healthy Fats**: Healthy fats are crucial for hormone production, brain health, and absorbing fat-soluble vitamins (A, D, E,

and K). They also keep you full and satisfied, reducing the urge to snack. Focus on sources like avocados, nuts, seeds, olive oil, and fatty fish.

3. **Choose Complex Carbohydrates**: While low-carb diets are popular, especially in fasting communities, carbohydrates are still an important part of a balanced diet. Opt for complex carbs that are high in fibre and low on the glycaemic index, such as vegetables, whole grains, and legumes. These will provide sustained energy without causing blood sugar spikes.

4. **Don't Forget Fibre**: Fibre is often overlooked but is essential for digestive health, blood sugar control, and satiety. Ensure your meals include fibre-rich foods like vegetables, fruits, nuts, seeds, and whole grains.

5. **Timing Matters**: When fasting, the timing of your meals can impact how well your body utilises macronutrients. Breaking your fast with a balanced meal that includes all three macronutrients (protein, fat, and carbs) helps stabilise blood sugar and prepares your body for the next fasting period.

Understanding why we crave certain foods, and the importance of nutrient-rich eating empowers you to make better choices. By balancing your macronutrients—especially during fasting—you can keep cravings at bay, maintain energy levels, and support your overall health. The key is to listen to your body, provide it with what it truly needs, and approach you're eating habits with mindfulness and intention.

Chapter 15: Mindset and Psychological Aspects

Staying Motivated and the Power of Habits

Success with intermittent fasting—or any significant lifestyle change—doesn't just hinge on what you do; it's also deeply rooted in how you think. While the physical benefits of fasting are undeniable, the true power lies in shifting your mindset. In this section, we'll explore how adopting the right mindset, focusing on identity-based habits, and rewarding yourself throughout the journey can lead to lasting transformation.

The Power of Habits: Identity-Based Transformation

Habits are the building blocks of our daily lives. They shape our behaviours, our decisions, and ultimately, our results. However, **the key to developing habits that stick lies not in what you do, but in who you believe you are.** This concept, known as identity-based habits, is transformative because it focuses on becoming the type of person who naturally embodies the habits you seek.

Instead of setting a goal to "lose weight" or "stick to intermittent fasting," shift your focus to the type of person you want to become. For example, rather than saying, "I want to lose 20 pounds," try saying, "I am someone who prioritises health and well-being." When you believe you are this person, your actions will naturally align with that identity.

Believing You Are Already There
A powerful aspect of this mindset shift is believing that you already are the person you aspire to be—even before the evidence shows it. When you start to act like the person who is fit, healthy, and disciplined, you begin to make choices that reflect that identity. This belief isn't about faking it until you make it; it's about embodying the qualities of the person you are becoming, which in turn leads to real, tangible change.

For example, if you see yourself as someone who is disciplined and mindful, you're more likely to stick to your fasting schedule, choose nutritious foods, and resist the temptation to overeat. Over time, these consistent actions reinforce your new identity, making the change feel natural and sustainable.

Reinforcing Habits with Rewards
Every transformational journey has its ups and downs, and staying motivated is key. One effective way to maintain momentum is to reward yourself for progress—no matter how small. Rewards don't have to be extravagant; they can be as simple as taking time to enjoy a favourite activity, buying yourself something special, or acknowledging your progress with a positive affirmation.

The key is to link these rewards to the new identity you're cultivating. For instance, if you've successfully completed a week of fasting, reward yourself with something that aligns with your health goals, like a new book on wellness, a beautiful candle or a relaxing day at the spa. These rewards help to reinforce the positive behaviours and keep you focused on the bigger picture.

It's important to note that rewards shouldn't be counterproductive. For instance, rewarding yourself with unhealthy food can sabotage your progress. Instead, **choose rewards that support your long-term goals** and reinforce your identity as a person who values health and well-being.

Overcoming Setbacks with a Growth Mindset
Even with the best intentions, setbacks are inevitable. How you respond to them makes all the difference. Adopting a growth mindset—where challenges are seen as opportunities to learn rather than failures—can help you stay on track. When faced with a setback, ask yourself: "What can I learn from this experience?" and "How can I use this to improve?" For example, if you break your fast earlier than planned or indulge in a craving, don't dwell on it. Instead, reflect on what led to that decision and how you can better prepare next time. This approach allows you to grow stronger with each challenge, rather than getting discouraged and giving up

Overcoming Emotional Eating

Addressing emotional eating requires a nuanced approach that goes beyond simply changing dietary habits. It involves a deep dive into the psychological triggers that drive food choices, and the emotional responses tied to eating. Recognising and understanding these triggers is crucial for developing healthier coping mechanisms. Techniques such as mindfulness, cognitive-behavioural strategies, and emotional awareness can help individuals identify and manage the underlying emotions that lead to overeating or unhealthy food choices.

Celebrating Small Wins

Equally important is the practice of celebrating small wins along the journey to better health.
Acknowledging and rewarding progress, no matter how incremental, fosters a positive mindset and reinforces commitment to long-term goals.
Celebrations of small victories, whether it's resisting a temptation, making a nutritious choice, or sticking to a new routine, help build confidence and motivation. By shifting focus from perfection to progress, individuals can cultivate a more compassionate relationship with themselves and their eating habits, paving the way for sustainable and rewarding changes.
Transformation is a journey, not a destination.
Along the way, it's essential to celebrate the small victories that lead to bigger changes. Each successful day of fasting, each healthy choice, and each positive affirmation is a win that should be acknowledged. These small wins accumulate, building confidence and reinforcing the belief that you are indeed the person you aspire to be.
Consider keeping a journal to track your progress and note the small wins. Reflecting on how far you've come, even when progress seems slow, can provide the motivation you need to keep going.

The journey to better health through intermittent fasting is as much about mindset as it is about action. By embracing the power of habits, believing in your identity as a healthy and disciplined person, and rewarding yourself along the way, you create a foundation for lasting change. Remember, you already are the person you want to become; now it's just a matter of letting that identity guide your actions, day by day.

Chapter 16: Long-Term Sustainability and Lifestyle Integration

Integrating Fasting into Everyday Life

Embarking on a journey toward improved health through fasting, mindful eating, and whole foods is a significant step, but the key to long-term success lies in making these practices a natural part of your daily routine. To integrate fasting seamlessly into your life, start by aligning your fasting schedules with your personal and professional commitments. Whether it's coordinating with work, family meals, or social events, choose a fasting method that complements your lifestyle. Begin with a manageable approach and gradually adapt it as needed, ensuring that fasting becomes an effortless and sustainable part of your day-to-day activities.

Adjusting Your Fasting Routine Over Time

As life evolves, so should your fasting routine. Periodically reassess your fasting schedule to ensure it aligns with any changes in your health, activity levels, or stress. Flexibility is essential—some days may require shorter fasts, while others might accommodate longer ones. For women, hormonal fluctuations throughout the menstrual cycle can impact energy levels and hunger, necessitating adjustments to fasting length or food choices. Stay adaptable and be willing to modify your fasting approach to better suit your changing needs and circumstances, helping maintain both effectiveness and sustainability.

How to Maintain Your Results

Embarking on a journey toward improved health through fasting, mindful eating, and whole foods is a powerful step, but the true challenge lies in maintaining these habits for the long haul. Sustainability is key to ensuring that the progress you've made isn't just temporary but becomes a lasting part of your lifestyle. Here's how to integrate these practices seamlessly into your daily life, ensuring they become second nature.

Shift Your Mindset: It's a Lifestyle, Not a Diet

One of the most important elements of long-term success is shifting your mindset from short-term dieting to embracing a holistic lifestyle. Diets often feel restrictive and temporary, leading to the infamous yo-yo effect where lost weight is quickly regained. Instead, view your approach as a permanent change, focusing on how these habits enhance your health, energy, and overall well-being.

By adopting the mindset that this is a lifestyle—one that prioritises nourishing your body, honouring your hunger signals, and treating food as fuel—you can create a sustainable approach to eating that doesn't feel like a sacrifice.

Flexibility is Key

Life is dynamic, and so should be your approach to health. While consistency is important, allowing for flexibility ensures you can adapt to life's changes without feeling guilty or derailed. Whether it's a special occasion, a holiday, or a busy week, recognise that it's okay to adjust your routine. If you've embraced fasting, for instance, some days may call for shorter fasts, while others might involve a longer fast. The same goes for your food choices—aim for balance rather than perfection.

For those with a menstrual cycle, flexibility is particularly important. Hormonal fluctuations can impact energy levels, hunger, and overall well-being, making it necessary to adjust the length of fasts or types of foods consumed at different times of the month. Listening to your body and being adaptable will support long-term adherence to your healthy lifestyle.

Focus on the Journey, Not Just the Destination
Achieving your health goals is important, but it's equally crucial to find joy in the journey. Celebrate small victories, like resisting a craving, trying a new recipe, or completing a successful fast. These moments build momentum and reinforce your commitment. Recognise that setbacks are a natural part of the process. Instead of viewing them as failures, see them as opportunities to learn, adjust, and keep moving forward.

Build a Supportive Environment
Your environment plays a significant role in your ability to sustain healthy habits. Surround yourself with people who understand and support your goals. This might mean involving family members, finding a community of like-minded individuals, or working with a coach or nutritionist. Additionally, set up your home in a way that supports your new lifestyle. Keep your kitchen stocked with healthy foods, minimise temptations, and create a routine that encourages mindfulness around meals and fasting.

Prioritise Self-Care and Stress Management
Sustainability isn't just about food; it's also about managing stress and prioritising self-care. Chronic stress can derail even the best intentions, leading to emotional eating, disrupted sleep, and decreased motivation. Incorporate stress management practices such as mindfulness, meditation, yoga, or regular physical activity into your routine. Taking care of your mental and emotional health is just as important as what you eat.

Continuous Learning and Adaptation
The journey toward better health is ongoing, and so is your learning. Stay curious and open to new information. As science evolves, so too might your approach. What worked well for you initially might need adjustment as your body and circumstances change. Keep refining your practices, trying new recipes, experimenting with different fasting protocols, and staying informed about the latest research. Consider reading books, following credible experts, or listening to podcasts that align with your health philosophy. This ongoing education will keep you engaged and motivated, helping you avoid stagnation.

Reward Yourself Along the Way
Finally, don't forget to reward yourself for your efforts. Rewards can be a powerful motivator and a way to reinforce positive behaviour. However, it's important to choose rewards that align with your health goals. For instance, instead of celebrating with a sugary treat, consider rewarding yourself with a relaxing massage, a new kitchen gadget, or a day trip to a place you love. Celebrating your progress reminds you of how far you've come and keeps you focused on the path ahead.

Sustaining a healthy lifestyle is about more than just willpower; it's about creating a supportive environment, embracing flexibility, and finding joy in the process. By integrating these practices into your daily life, you can build a foundation that not only helps you achieve your goals but also supports your health and well-being for years to come. Remember, this is a lifelong journey. Embrace the changes, be kind to yourself, and enjoy the rewards of a healthier, happier you.

Chapter 17: Top 10 Tips for Successful Intermittent Fasting and Improved Health

Intermittent fasting is a powerful tool for weight loss and overall health, but like any approach, it works best when combined with smart strategies. Here are ten tips to help you get the most out of your fasting journey:

Top 10 Tips

1. Set a Consistent Eating Window, but Be Flexible

Consistency is key, but it's also important to vary your fasting routine, especially for those with a menstrual cycle. Hormonal fluctuations can affect how your body responds to fasting, so consider adjusting the length of your fasts throughout the month. For instance, during the luteal phase (the week or two before your period), shorter fasts or increased caloric intake might be beneficial to avoid unnecessary stress on your body.

2. Stay Hydrated

Water is your best friend during fasting. Staying well-hydrated helps curb hunger, flush out toxins, and keeps you feeling energised. Herbal teas, black coffee, and electrolyte-rich beverages (without added sugars) can also be helpful but avoid any drinks that could break your fast.

3. Manage Cravings with Smart Strategies

Cravings are normal, especially when you first start fasting. When they strike, distract yourself with a quick walk, drink a glass of water, or engage in a non-food activity. Often, cravings are more psychological than physical—so give them time to pass. For those with a menstrual cycle, be mindful that cravings might increase at certain times of the month; plan your fasting schedule and meals accordingly.

4. Prioritise Whole, Unprocessed Foods
During your eating window, focus on whole foods that are nutrient-dense and satisfying. Eliminate ultra-processed foods (UPFs), bad oils (like trans fats and highly refined vegetable oils), and refined sugars. These foods spike insulin levels and promote fat storage, counteracting the benefits of fasting.

5. Don't Overcomplicate Your Meals
Intermittent fasting doesn't require special foods or complicated meal plans. Keep it simple with balanced meals that include lean proteins, healthy fats, and plenty of vegetables. The goal is to nourish your body with real food, not to obsess over calorie counting.

6. Listen to Your Body and Adjust Fasting Lengths
Pay attention to how your body responds to different fasting schedules and food choices. Varying the length of your fasts can help prevent metabolic slowdown and support hormonal balance. For example, incorporate longer fasts (such as 24 or 36 hours) occasionally, but listen to your body, especially during different phases of the menstrual cycle, and adjust as needed.

7. Exercise Wisely

While exercise is great for overall health, **weight loss with intermittent fasting isn't dependent on working out.** Focus on maintaining an active lifestyle with activities you enjoy, such as walking, yoga, or strength training. Exercise can enhance the benefits of fasting, but it's not the primary driver of fat loss— diet and fasting are. On days when you extend your fasting window or are experiencing hormonal changes, consider lighter or restorative exercises.

8. Break Your Fast Mindfully
When it's time to break your fast, start with a light meal that's easy to digest. Avoid jumping straight into heavy or carb-laden meals, as this can cause blood sugar spikes and undo some of the fasting benefits.

9. Practice Patience and Self-Compassion
Intermittent fasting is a long-term lifestyle change, not a quick fix. Be patient with yourself as your body adapts, and don't get discouraged by setbacks. Celebrate small victories and remember that progress is more important than perfection. For those with a menstrual cycle, understand that some months may feel easier than others—be gentle with yourself and adjust your approach accordingly.

10. Focus on the Bigger Picture
Health is about more than just losing weight. Intermittent fasting can improve your metabolic health, enhance mental clarity, and increase longevity. Keep these broader benefits in mind as you continue your journey and let them motivate you to stay consistent. Recognise that varying your fasting routine can optimise these benefits and support long-term success.

Key Do's and Don'ts for Intermittent Fasting

- **Do** keep your fasting window consistent but allow flexibility for hormonal cycles.
- **Do** stay hydrated and manage cravings with smart strategies.
- **Do** prioritise whole, unprocessed foods during your eating window.
- **Do** listen to your body, adjust fasting lengths, and vary your routine for better results.
- **Don't** overcomplicate your meals—focus on balanced, simple nutrition.
- **Don't** rely on exercise alone for weight loss—diet and fasting are key.
- **Don't** break your fast with heavy or sugary foods.
- **Don't** rush the process—be patient and kind to yourself, especially during different phases of your menstrual cycle.

Chapter 18: Conclusion

Reflecting on the Journey

As I look back on my journey with intermittent fasting, it's clear that this lifestyle change has been nothing short of transformative. From my initial struggles with weight management to the profound improvements in my health and well-being, intermittent fasting has provided me with a renewed sense of vitality and balance and a sense that I'm in control.

After years of chasing fleeting diet trends and battling frustration, discovering intermittent fasting was a turning point. The gradual adjustments, from the 16:8 method to exploring longer fasts, allowed me to reconnect with my body's natural rhythms and achieve sustainable results. The unexpected benefits, such as improved sleep quality, increased energy levels, and significant weight loss, have surpassed my expectations.

What stands out the most is the shift in my relationship with food. No longer driven by constant cravings or the cycle of deprivation and reward, then guilt, I now approach eating with mindfulness and satisfaction. My husband's parallel experience with intermittent fasting further reinforced the effectiveness and adaptability of this approach. Together, we navigated the challenges and celebrated the victories, finding a healthier and more harmonious way of living.

This journey has not only transformed our bodies but has also enriched our lives with a sense of accomplishment and well-being that we hadn't anticipated. Intermittent fasting has shown us that maintaining a healthy weight is achievable with the right mindset and approach, proving that it's never too late to make meaningful changes.

Encouragement for Readers: You Can Do This Too

To anyone reading this book who might be feeling overwhelmed or sceptical, I want to offer a message of hope and encouragement: You can do this too. The path to better health doesn't have to be daunting or unattainable. If you've struggled with weight management or dietary frustrations, know that intermittent fasting can be a powerful tool to help you achieve your goals.

Start with small, manageable steps and gradually build your fasting routine. Be patient with yourself and embrace the journey as a learning experience. Remember that it's not just about the numbers on a scale but about the holistic improvements in your energy, mood, and overall health.

Intermittent fasting is not a one-size-fits-all solution, but it offers a flexible framework that can be tailored to fit your lifestyle. Listen to your body, adjust as needed, and don't be afraid to explore different fasting styles to find what works best for you.

Most importantly, stay motivated and believe in your ability to succeed. The benefits you can achieve are worth the effort, and the positive changes you'll experience will be a testament to your commitment and perseverance. As you embark on or continue your own journey with intermittent fasting, remember that you have the power to transform your health and well-being.

Thank you for joining me on this journey. I hope that my experiences and insights have provided you with the inspiration and practical guidance you need to make intermittent fasting a part of your life. Here's to your health, your vitality, and the incredible possibilities that lie ahead.

Resources and Further Reading

Recommended Books

Books:

- Fast Like a Girl: A Woman's Guide to Using the Healing Power of Fasting to Burn Fat, Boost Energy, and Balance Hormones – Dr. Mindy Pelz
- The Menopause Reset: Get Rid of Your Symptoms and Feel Like Your Younger Self Again – Dr. Mindy Pelz
- It's Not a Diet: The No Cravings, No Willpower Way to Get Lean and Happy for Good – Davinia Taylor
- Hack Your Hormones: Effortless Weight Loss. Better Focus. Deeper Sleep. More Energy – Davinia Taylor
- Ultra-Processed People: Why Do We All Eat Stuff That Isn't Food...and Why Can't We Stop? - Chris van Tulleken
- Glucose Revolution: The life-changing power of balancing your blood sugar - Jessie Inchauspé
- Atomic Habits - James Clear
- The Power of Habit - Charles Duhigg

Useful Websites and Communities

https://drmindypelz.com/
https://www.willpowders.com/
For Fats Sake Club! Facebook group brought to you by Davinia Taylor & Will Powders

Acknowledgments

I want to extend my heartfelt gratitude to my incredible husband, Simon, whose unwavering support has made this journey possible. Your encouragement has been a guiding light, and your belief in this project has been invaluable.

To our amazing children, Max and Millie, your constant enthusiasm and encouragement have been a wellspring of motivation. Your love and presence, even when we're not together, remind me daily of what truly matters and keep me focused on the path ahead.

I am also deeply grateful to the experts who have profoundly influenced my journey. Dr. Mindy Pelz, your pioneering work has been a beacon of knowledge and inspiration. Davinia Taylor, your enthusiasm and personal insights have been both enlightening and empowering. And Chris van Tulleken, your expertise and perspectives around the pervasive UPF industry have opened my eyes and broadened my understanding in ways I could not have achieved alone.

Thank you all for your invaluable contributions. This book reflects the collective wisdom and support I have received along the way. Here's to many more years of health, happiness, and continued learning together. With sincere thanks,

Allison

About the Author

Allison is a health enthusiast, writer, and advocate for sustainable lifestyle changes. With over 20 years of personal experience in exploring and refining healthy living practices, Allison combines a deep understanding of the importance of nutrition, fitness, and behavioural psychology to help others achieve lasting well-being.

Personal Journey to Health

Like many people, Allison's weight loss journey was not linear. After decades of struggling with various diets, and the emotional toll of unmet goals, Allison discovered intermittent fasting—a method that not only transformed her physical health but also reshaped her approach to food, mindset, and self-care.

Drawing from personal experience, Allison has spent recent years researching the science behind intermittent fasting, delving into its benefits, and understanding its impact on long-term health. This book is a culmination of that journey—a blend of personal insights, practical advice, and evidence-based research to guide readers on their own path to health.

Educational Background and Research

Allison's commitment to better understanding the science of intermittent fasting led to an extensive review of academic literature and research studies. This foundation includes studies on metabolism, insulin regulation, autophagy, and the psychological aspects of habit formation. Key references that have informed the approach in this book include:

- **Metabolic Benefits**: Research by Dr. Jason Fung, a nephrologist and author, on the role of insulin resistance and the effectiveness of fasting in reversing type 2 diabetes, has significantly influenced Allison's understanding of how intermittent fasting impacts metabolism and fat loss.
- **Autophagy and Cellular Health**: The groundbreaking work of Dr. Yoshinori Ohsumi, who won the Nobel Prise in Physiology or Medicine in 2016 for his discoveries on autophagy, provides the scientific backing for the cellular renewal benefits of fasting discussed in this book.
- **Behavioural Science and Habits**: Insights from James Clear's *Atomic Habits* and Charles Duhigg's *The Power of Habit* have shaped Allison's approach to habit formation, particularly the concept of identity-based habits and the power of small wins in driving long-term change.
- **Longevity and Hormonal Health**: Studies on fasting's impact on longevity, such as the work published in *Cell Metabolism* by Dr. Valter Longo, have provided crucial insights into how intermittent fasting can improve not just weight loss, but overall health and longevity.

Mission and Vision

Allison Butnick is dedicated to helping others achieve lasting health by demystifying intermittent fasting and making it accessible to everyone, regardless of their starting point. Through this book, Allison aims to empower readers to take control of their health, not just through dietary changes, but by fostering a positive mindset, building sustainable habits, and embracing a lifestyle that honours both body and mind.

When not writing or researching, Allison runs a life and career coaching company and enjoys cooking healthy meals, practicing yoga and mindfulness.

Connect with Allison

To contact Allison about her work, insights on health and wellness, and upcoming projects email allison@shine-now.co.uk.

Copyright Page

Title: From Blaming Myself to Finding the Truth: How Intermittent Fasting Changed My Life

Printed in Great Britain
by Amazon

46458273R00059